where did you go?

where
did
you
go?

A Life-Changing Journey
to Connect with
Those We've Lost

CHRISTINA RASMUSSEN

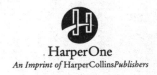

HarperOne
An Imprint of HarperCollinsPublishers

HarperOne

WHERE DID YOU GO? Copyright © 2018 by Christina Rasmussen.
All rights reserved. Printed in the United States of America. No part of this
book may be used or reproduced in any manner whatsoever without written
permission except in the case of brief quotations embodied in critical articles
and reviews. For information, address HarperCollins Publishers,
195 Broadway, New York, NY 10007.

HarperCollins books may be purchased for educational, business, or sales
promotional use. For information, please email the Special Markets Department
at SPsales@harpercollins.com.

FIRST EDITION

Designed by Yvonne Chan

Library of Congress Cataloging-in-Publication Data is available upon request.

ISBN 978-0-06-268962-7

18 19 20 21 22 LSC 10 9 8 7 6 5 4 3 2 1

Bjarne, may you find yourself in other universes living with soulmates who love you as much as we do.

contents

introduction

Everything we call real is made of things
that cannot be regarded as real.
—NIELS BOHR, NOBEL PRIZE–WINNING PHYSICIST

It can be difficult to believe in the *afterlife* if we haven't had our own direct encounters with that world. All we're really left with are mere descriptions of it, based on two-thousand-year-old religious texts that may feel far removed from our modern world, or accounts of mystical journeys that seem to happen to just a special few. For many of us, without that direct evidence of where our loved ones have gone, our minds are unable to grasp the possibility of a world we cannot see, of a world beyond this one. Our resistance to an expanded awareness is reinforced by what *seems* like science's privileging of the empirical above all else: the world is three-dimensional, and nothing exists beyond it.

But the fact is, the essence of who we are, our individual consciousness, continues after death. There is indeed a world beyond this one. It's hidden. Our loved ones have gone there, and we can, too. Without dying. We can access it, regardless of our religious beliefs or lack of any mystical abilities.

This guidebook will help you experience it. It will break down the science about life after life in accessible language that will allow you to believe in the continuation of consciousness. It will help you believe that the people we've loved and lost aren't gone. They're part of the hidden reality that we, too, are a part of, just not aware of it.

I'm hoping this book will change the way you grieve and the way you come back to life after loss. I believe if you knew that death was not the end for the person you lost you would live your life more fully. With zest. With boldness. Yes, you would still miss that person and mourn the loss, but the knowledge that you can connect with their consciousness would make your journey back to living life fully a little easier. And if you haven't lost someone you love, but have a fear of dying or are curious about what comes next so you can live to your true potential, this book is also for you.

When a loved one dies, we can open a door between this world and the next. It only closes when we don't look for it, when we don't observe it, and when we don't believe it's there. When we walk through this door, we go on a journey to an invisible place. I have named that place the Temple World.

Typically, in the weeks and months following the death of our beloveds, we're too emotionally distraught to step through that door in our consciousness. After, when we reclaim our lives and come back to an everyday routine, we doubt that world exists. Even if we're religious, I believe there can be doubt. We want to believe and have faith in that world—both to know that our loved ones are okay, and that we, too, will be okay after we die—but our logical brain fights that.

Our logical brain exists and operates in the third dimension—the dimension you're experiencing right now—and shuts down anything beyond it. But once you have gathered your strength after a loss and allowed life back into your everyday routine, the Temple World is there waiting for you to observe it, to consciously be part of it. I know you've sensed this world after losing your loved one—maybe you felt your loved one's hand on your shoulder, heard soothing words in your mind, or even saw that person for a brief moment.

I wrote this book to help you find the door to the Temple World and give yourself permission to look for it, observe it, and bring it into your reality. The door to this world is right here next to you; it's anywhere you're able to close your eyes and tap into the hidden reality I will introduce you to. I know your brain will try to tell you there is no other world. But once you can guide it to that world, you'll be led to a place you can be a part of every single day if you wish. Once there, you'll meet with the people you lost and experience a sense of joy and peace. You will also feel a sense of wholeness and unity with the bigger cosmos that leaves you speechless. I want to help you find your footing there and assist you in taking one step farther in your life after loss. I call this step the Temple Journey.

As you're doing the exercises of this book, you'll likely find that you feel part human, part "something else"—which is your true essence, without the confines of your body. And it will feel uncomfortable at first. I'm going to help you get used to that. My goal is that when you get to the last page of this book, you will feel that it's normal to talk to the people you lost and to connect with the hidden invisible world that exists all around you. And because you'll be the one taking the journey and connecting directly with your loved ones—not receiving information through a psychic or a medium—you might just gather enough proof and develop a strong enough sense of knowing to deeply believe that death isn't the end and the people you lost are only a dimension away. I wouldn't ask you to go anywhere I haven't been myself. I had to find tools and methods of seeing the invisible world without "having the gift." But I've discovered that we all have the gift of consciousness and we all can tap into a heightened awareness that can serve in nearly the same way.

As you have gathered by now, the purpose of this book is not to analyze visions of ghosts or discuss mediums who transmit messages from another dimension. While I appreciate their powers, and the experiences those powers open to them, this book is about *our* experiences—yours and mine, everyday people. This book is about giving you permission to believe in your own abilities. It's about experiencing life beyond our physical reality, beyond the 3-D world that's only a tiny part of what we call reality. It's for those of us who wish to make journeying beyond our physical reality an everyday experience—normal, natural, and not at all scary. Visiting nonphysical realms is actually natural, rather than supernatural. Those visits are so full of healing, immense peace, awe, and deepened intuition that you begin to understand life and death a little better. Access to that understanding and that seemingly invisible world is our birthright.

I am inviting you to come along on this journey with me. Say yes to revealing an unseen energetic layer that surrounds us, that we're actually a part of. Our soul yearns to witness and experience this nonphysical layer, not only for us to fully heal, but also to make the absolute most of our lives.

How to Use This Book

This book is set up so you read a new chapter each week, in chronological order. With the exception of the last chapter, each chapter focuses on a new journey within the Temple World. For instance, the first journey, called the Door (chapter 3 in this book), takes you on the crossing into the Temple World, where you'll find the person you've lost and/or those who come to help guide you.

You'll take each chapter's journey for ten minutes or so a day every day for one week. If you need to spend an extra week on a particular journey, that's fine. However, I don't recommend you spend less than one week on each journey—you'll need that time to trust in your experience. On these journeys, you'll gain knowledge about the universe, energy, light, and your own consciousness. Each journey will expand your awareness and change your life in your day-to-day world. And if you wish to read the whole book in one go, that's okay too. Just rest when you need to. And pace yourself.

You'll also have the choice to journey with a group of people who are all reading the book together. In the Resources section at the back of this book you'll find information about how to find or set up these groups. Each chapter also contains tools to use on your journey, such as sounds and vibrations, that you'll download from the Life Reentry Institute website. You'll find the link in the Resources section as well.

As you go farther on the Temple Journey you'll begin to understand that our physical existence on Earth is only one part of who we are. You'll experience what we know as time in an entirely new way. Einstein proved that time is relative, not absolute. Past, present, and future occur simultaneously. Within the Temple World, the construct of time doesn't exist. To imagine what that's like, just think how a smell or a song can transport you right to a specific moment in time. Many of the students I've taken on this journey have seen events in their current life through a different filter—more perceptive, detached, loving—that offers greater understanding of an event. Some see future events in great detail, which often gives them an understanding to better navigate the present in their day-to-day lives.

On this journey you'll experience this collapse of time as we know it, the time we've created as a species to make sense of our 3-D reality. You'll learn that you can visit your beloved who's died in this world instead of having to passively wait for (or becoming freaked out by) that person popping in on you.

Finally, you get to partner with the universe; communicate with the loved ones you've lost from this world; dance with the Field, the web of energy that surrounds us all and connects everyone and everything; and become one with what I have called your Super Watcher, who is your divinity, your higher self, your cosmic self. This world we live in is not the only world in existence, but our brain makes us believe there are no other worlds. No other dimensions. No other ways to live.

We'll change all that. Together. Here's to a journey unlike any other. Here's to an experience that brings together science, faith, religion, and, above all, God, Source, the Universe, Spirit—whichever term you prefer for divine consciousness. A journey we're all on, even if we don't realize it yet. Open yourself to experiencing what you've been told can't be experienced. Let go of the old beliefs, the advice, the containers you built to stow your loss and compartmentalize your life. Let it all spill out. All I ask you to do is go through the Door.

where did you go?

I don't want to believe. I want to know.

—CARL SAGAN

I created the Temple World because when I was just thirty-four, my husband, whom I loved deeply, died. In this world, he was gone forever, existing only in photos, home videos, and our memories—but I couldn't accept that he no longer existed at all. He had to be *somewhere* in the universe. What if, after his three-and-a-half-year battle with colon cancer, he was at peace in another world, one I could not see? I needed to know. I needed to know he was okay.

So I became a reporter of the invisible world—the world on the other side of the Door between life and death. A finder of words required to make these worlds real for both me and you. "Where did you go?" was the first question I asked Bjarne, wherever he was, after I left the hospital, walked into what had been our bedroom, and closed the door behind me. In my mind, I asked this question thousands of times. And even when I reentered and rebuilt my life, that one question persisted: *Where did you go?* By going on this journey, I found him.

This was definitely not a journey I *wanted* to go on. For three and a half years, I held on to the hope and belief that he would live longer, but there was no stopping the cancer. The journey of searching for my husband began the day he died. I knew then that my life was about to change irrevocably, but I didn't understand all that would encompass.

I remember that day clearly. Bjarne had been in the hospital for ten days. Every one of those days I'd sat on the side of his hospital bed, legs curled under me, witnessing cancer hijack his body until I hardly recognized him. Sunken cheekbones. Blond hair gone dark. Pale skin, almost beige, matching the hospital walls. His eyes still blue, but the kind of blue you find in the middle of the ocean. Dusky. Those ten days were truly unbearable.

Late in the morning of the tenth day, it was clear that the end was very close. That's when the doctors had started to administer the coma-inducing drugs to help with his breathing, and Bjarne turned to me and very quietly said, "Bring the kids. It's time." I called my mom to bring the girls as soon as possible. An hour later, the girls stormed into the room and jumped on their dad's bed. I quietly moved out of their way. "Hi, Daddy," our older daughter said, climbing onto his chest. Our younger followed. Under the oxygen mask, his mouth widened into a grin, smiling at his girls. He started singing and they joined him. His voice, a distant echo of what it once was, brought back the nights he'd spent singing with the girls while putting them to bed. For a few short seconds, I forgot where we were, and a smile sneaked in. He'd been holding on to all his energy for this moment.

After a few minutes, I could see he was getting tired, his eyes starting to close.

"Girls," I said, placing my hands on their backs, "it's time to say good-bye to Daddy."

"Mommy, no," my older daughter said. "Not yet."

"Daddy needs to sleep again, love," I said, then asked her to give him a kiss.

The girls kissed their dad good-bye. They didn't know it would be for the last time. But he did. He opened his eyes once again, waved, and gave them his biggest smile.

When the girls left, I leaned over and placed my head on top of his, so he could see me if he opened his eyes. I lay there, holding his hand, my body half on the bed, half off. The morphine drip had started to work.

"Bjarne, it's my turn to say good-bye now," I said in my quietest voice. I waited for a response. Nothing. Then he turned his head away from me. He'd spent all his energy on the girls and I couldn't help but feel robbed of my moment with him. I leaned over him again, trying to get his attention one more time.

"My love. It's my turn to say good-bye now," I whispered, a little louder this time. No response. No eye movement. No hand squeezing. The hiss of the oxygen machine, the loud whispering of the nurses and doctors in the hall—everything ear-splitting. For nearly four years, since his cancer diagnosis, I had pictured the moment when we'd say good-bye. It wasn't turning out the way I'd imagined. I'd always thought we'd hug for hours. Instead, I was begging for a nod and he was silently begging for the end.

A few hours went by quietly. Nurses, family, and friends came into and out of the room. Suddenly, Bjarne sat up, started muttering, and reached toward something only he could see. I leaped off the bed, tried to talk to him, tried to help. His eyes slid past me. I grabbed his arm, but he didn't flinch. For the first time in our lives together, he looked at me, but he didn't know me. I deeply wanted to see what he was seeing and share the moment with him. But he was going somewhere else, somewhere the girls and I couldn't follow. I leaned closer to hear what he was saying but couldn't quite make it out. He was calling to someone, over and over. Someone who wasn't me.

In the midst of this, a nurse hurried in. "Let me see what's going on here," she said. "He's not supposed to be able to sit up, or even be awake." She quickly attached a new bag of medicine to his IV and helped him lie back down, as though to erase the moment she couldn't explain. *What was she doing?* I wasn't finished trying to get his attention, trying to bring him back to me. Almost immediately, he lapsed into sleep, and the room was quiet once again. "That should do it," she said, and looked at me as if we both had the same goal—to hurry his dying along.

Night came. I never left the room. The pale walls now held an added dimension of gray. From the stale-smelling bag of clothes and toiletries I'd brought to the hospital, I grabbed a pair of leggings. I walked to the corner of the room and pulled them on quickly, before anyone could walk into the room. I'd just made it back to the bed when someone knocked gently on the door. The knock sounded different from usual—certain, but quiet. The doctors would knock loudly, then barge in before I could respond.

"Come on in," I said.

The door opened. It was the oncology nurse, Robin, who'd been with us for the past three and a half years. Since the diagnosis, she'd been a member of our medical team and a part of our journey. She put her hand on my husband's head. I knew she'd made this type of visit many times. There was a strength there I could draw on. Over the years, I'd always been comforted by that strength when she was in the treatment room. "I want to show you something, "she said and bent down closer to my husband's face.

"Hi there, Bjarne," she said. "It's Robin." She spoke quite loudly, louder than my prior attempts. To my surprise, as soon as she spoke to him, he mumbled something back to her. "You see? He can hear you," she said, smiling. "You can tell him whatever you want, and he'll hear you." She straightened, turning to leave.

"But wait, isn't he in a coma?" I got up from the bed to stand beside her.

"Yes, he is, but he can hear you, me, and everything going on around him. There are some things we can't understand. This is one of them." She patted my hand.

As soon as she left, I turned to my husband. I put my hands on either side of his head and moved as close to him as I could. "I love you," I said loudly, and he responded, mumbling a word I couldn't quite understand. It sounded like "Mmmmm," as if he wanted me to know he could hear me. I felt a jolt of joy rise within me, even though I knew it was still the end. Every five minutes I said the words to him. "I love you." Every time he responded. "Mmmmm." He kept responding all the way to his last breath.

"I love you," I said for the last time.

"Mmmmm," he said, and took his last breath in, then out. He was gone.

I actually looked up to see if I could see Bjarne hovering above. I was looking for his soul but saw only the ceiling with the ugly fluorescent light. I looked around me and there was nothing there. Looked at him, and his body seemed empty. He could no longer hear me. He wasn't coming back.

In the days, weeks, and months that followed Bjarne's death, I swung between mind-numbing grief and an insatiable search for him, for his essence. One moment I was painfully sad, the next moment I was hunting for his ghost, spirit body, soul—anything that was him.

Even though I'd been brought up Greek Orthodox, my religious background didn't help me. It actually deepened my doubts about what it really meant to me, my girls, and our life, that someone we loved was now in a place called heaven, or the afterlife. At the time, for me, the reality of the afterlife just wasn't plausible. I wasn't into the idea that Bjarne was now in heaven. Not in the traditional version of heaven anyway. I didn't care much about the usual expressions about the soul passing. I wasn't consoled by phrases like "He's with the angels now," or "He's no longer in pain." They maddened me.

I wanted facts. I wanted to *know* he'd gone somewhere else; hoping and imagining weren't enough. I wanted to know that even though he was dead here, he was alive there, wherever there was. I wanted to believe. I was desperate to know what had happened to him. In searching for answers, reading whatever books about this other world I could find became a nearly daily activity for me. I consulted gifted psychics, talked to priests, and listened to every story anyone wanted to share with me about his or her own experience with the afterlife. But I also searched for facts. God wasn't a fact for me during those days, or even during the years that followed. Don't get me wrong—I *wanted* to believe Bjarne was with God and the angels in heaven, or in another universe I knew nothing about; anything but dead. Not knowing that his consciousness had survived his physical death was breaking my heart. But I needed something concrete to hold on to. Something I could believe in.

The journey that started the day my husband died has been the most important journey of my life. I spent those first few years after his passing barely surviving. Living day in and day out inside a routine that took away my passion for life. A routine based on fear of the future and dictated by my ego's need to "protect" me by keeping me stuck in one place. I hated my life, my future, and every moment of every day. I was jealous of women whose husbands were still alive, jealous of parents taking their kids out for pancakes on a Sunday morning and living their perfect lives. I was a bitter, angry young widow. Dark thoughts filled my head, an ugly monster roaring. Not a pretty picture, and one I'm not proud of. But it's the truth.

The years went by. The searching and rote surviving continued. I discovered brain science and immersed myself in that world. Brain science was the only field at the time that gave me a sense of hope because it studied the brain and its finding a way out of the pain. I could do something with that, instead of just existing in a never-ending state of grief, "waiting," as so many books on griev-ing advised, "for time to heal me," while at the same time telling me that "grief is supposed to last forever." These two concepts made me furious because waiting for time to pass was not the way I wanted to spend my life. But that exact thing, this terrible advice I was given, fueled my mission to impact the world of grief with an action-oriented process. In 2010, based on what I'd learned about neuroscience, I developed my Life Reentry Model to help people find their way back to life after loss. I launched my blog Second Firsts. I quit the corporate job I'd taken a little more than a year after Bjarne's death.

During the next few years, I didn't just get my own life back, I helped thousands of others do the same. But still, there was always one part missing. I worked with so many people who continued to search for their beloveds—even after they had reclaimed their own lives; even when they were thriving. I, too, continued to search. In some way, it wasn't enough to find our way back to a good life; once we had started reentering our lives and could face such questions, we were hungry to discover where our loved ones had gone and where we would be going one day. I wanted to see what Bjarne saw in the hospital room when he came out of the coma with his arms up in the air. I wanted to feel what he felt. I wanted to visit him, wherever he had gone.

My girls, too, had been looking for their dad. "Mommy, do you think he's here with us right now?" they asked over the years—at a graduation, or on a birthday, or just before I put them to bed. They still ask. And I remind them of the amazing moments and dreams they experienced the first few years after their dad died.

Not long after Bjarne's death, my younger daughter, Isabel, gave me one of her drawings. "Mommy," she said proudly, holding a piece of paper in front of her, "look, I drew a picture of us." She pointed to each person in the picture. "Mommy, here's you. That's me. Here's Elina. And the ghost," she said, pointing at a fuzzy cloud hovering on the right side of the drawing.

"Who's the ghost?" I asked her in surprise.

"It's Daddy." She then jumped from my lap and went off to her room. As kids do.

I wanted to keep talking about the picture. I wished she'd say more. It felt so good that she was experiencing things I couldn't. And that she wasn't scared of these experiences, as I imagined I would be if I saw Bjarne hanging around. Kids want to know the truth and are open to it, more than we are. As open as I've become, as often as I talk to Bjarne, my girls talk to their dad even more. Even ten years after his passing, they seek him out. It's a deeply healing experience to connect with him from this plane and to have the certainty and the confidence to believe in the unseen that surrounds us. But it took me nearly eight years to get to that place of certainty and confidence.

The Next Chapter

I slowly started to pick up my very painful life. A new promotion at work. Some new friends. My heart started beating a little faster and life began to lighten. In 2010, four years after Bjarne died, I remarried. My new husband, Eric, and I merged our families. Three years later, Eric, our four girls, and I moved from the Boston area to Northern California. Our house on top of a hill provided a perfect place to watch the sun rise over the mountains every day. When I watched the sun rise, my soul took the deepest breath. The senses of peace and expansion were palpable. I felt them in my body, every cell filling with light and air.

One day during those first few months after we'd moved, I was sitting at the table on our deck, watching the sun rise, when I felt everything go quiet, and an incredible euphoria came over me. All I could hear were the birds. That feeling of joy was unlike anything I'd ever felt—as though time had stopped, and everything made sense. That was my first "peak experience," the term renowned humanist psychologist Abraham H. Maslow coined to describe moments of such transcendent joy that they are almost spiritual.[1] Peak experiences come to us suddenly, filling us with wonder and pure awe. We feel a connection with the world around us, a oneness with every living thing. Maslow discusses humankind's yearning for the magical and describes how these experiences help us connect with the invisible world around us. The woman sitting on my deck during that peak experience, calm, at peace, filled with joy, was very different from the terrified woman who'd lain on her bed each night with all the lights on, waiting to experience something outside her own reality. This felt more like an extension of me and a blending with the nature that surrounded me. It felt like a rebirth.

That morning, my door to the invisible world opened. After that, I felt that activation, that bliss, every day when I watched the sun rise, and every night when I walked outside and gazed at the stars. No matter what difficulties my day brought, I found my way back to that place of peace and connection at night and in the early morning, and felt recalibrated. I experienced a different kind of life reentry. I traveled to a place of heightened consciousness. Of course, I still had to do the work in the physical world, but the journey felt so much bigger, so much lighter, as if I had discovered a secret place that was so large it was hidden in plain sight, around us all.

In these experiences I was reminded that my desire to uncover the truth about life after life—about the persistence of consciousness after death—had never disappeared. I consumed all the books and articles on neuroscience, quantum physics, and particle physics that I could get my hands on. I read about consciousness surviving outside the body, alternate realities, multiple dimensions, stars, black holes, time—anything that would help me understand a nonreligious, nonmystical possibility of life after life.

The deeper into the theories I went, the more I realized how much our scientists already know about the universe. But these findings have not made their way to the masses. How much evidence we actually have that these other dimensions exist—from personal accounts to theories in quantum physics, to discoveries accepted as fact in the scientific community. I realized that we've gone far in our discoveries but not far in our experiences and certainly not far in the sharing of these discoveries.

One of the very first things we learned when our scientists started to study the invisible parts of the universe was that everything in the universe contains both wave *and* particle. But what are these you may wonder? How is that relevant to life beyond life? Well, you see, a wave is the movement of energy from one location to another. In quantum physics, a particle is a small mass, the tiniest thing you can imagine. A particle is matter; it occupies space, however small it is. When scientists discovered that all objects are made of both waves and particles, both energy and matter, they were taken by surprise. In other words, matter is energy. This book you are reading is energy. To me, the fact that everything is energy means that the invisible hidden reality, which I have named the Temple World, is made of the exact same elements as the chair you're sitting on. And if that's true, all that we experience in the seemingly invisible world of the quantum realm, the Temple World, is as concrete as the experiences in our 3-D reality. Ultimately, we're swimming in energy that looks like matter.

Scientists also learned that when waves are being observed, they can behave as particles. It seems as if everything is probable, in a constant state of change. Therefore, at certain points in time, every version of reality is probable. When we're inside the Temple World interacting with our beloved, seeing and experiencing a different version of reality, our own reality changes. Maybe we can't bring the people we lost back to the dimension we live and work in, but we can interact with them inside the sea of energy and together see a new life.

When I read about quantum entanglement, the idea that everything—at the smallest level—is forever connected, my heart sped. No matter how far two entangled particles are from each other, they can always affect the other. Einstein called it "spooky action at a distance." Here's why I got so excited: humans are made of atoms, and atoms are made of subatomic particles. When we entangle with other humans, with other particles, the way we entangled with our beloved, we are never ever separated. The person we lost is entangled with us and always will be.

Quantum physics portrays a murky reality—no time, no truly solid matter, nothing existing until we observe it. What we consider real—such as the objects that constitute our everyday environment—isn't so real after all. They're part of what Einstein called "illusion." We observe the illusion, the hologram, that creates realities. Stepping out of the illusion of the hologram also means that we step out of the illusion of death, which excited me enormously. But I get that it can be unsettling. Though Einstein refused to accept quantum physics because, as he said, "I like to think the moon is there even if I am not looking at it," I saw only possibilities.

If the moon exists only when we're looking at it, where is it when we're not? If our beloveds can't be seen, is it because we don't know how to see them? And if learning how to look and experience differently with those we lost is the key to communicating with them, then what are we waiting for? I had to find the bridge between the way we see reality now and seeing it differently. To peeling back the layers of our very complex reality and finding my way in. What was the bridge made of? How could everyone find their way there? And if reality is only real because of how our eyes and brain observe it, then what if we tried to observe without our eyes and brain? What if we could trick our brain to see and shut down our senses to experience?

After researching, reading, asking questions, and learning as much as I could from what science has been telling us I caught a glimpse of the bridge between the physical world we live in and the nonphysical world, a bridge that had always been there, available only, it seemed, to mystics and physicists. Only they knew the way to the bridge. Only they tread its boards. What map did they possess? What worlds were they seeing on the other side? In the afterlife? What is really the meaning of that word—"afterlife"? What takes place after our life? Fascinating as these books were, these scientists weren't showing us the way. They weren't telling us where they were going, how they got there. They were simply telling us what they were seeing or hearing when they got there.

These books were heady, idea-laden, removed from everyday experience. These books offered a window to what's possible but provided no way for me to incorporate that knowledge into my everyday life, no way to connect with what I could not see. No tips. I kept asking myself, *How do I take what I've learned about the complex reality our consciousness inhabits through the filter of our brains and use it for our own good and our own life after loss?*

In *Second Firsts*, I wrote of the gap between two worlds—the world before loss, and the one after. But in trying to build a bridge between yet another two worlds—the physical and the nonphysical—I faced another gap: the gap between the abstractions in the quantum physics and that of my own reality. Something large was missing. There was no visible bridge. A how to manual. A map. A step-by-step guide.

So, I began a new journey to bring this bridge forth, a bridge between the two worlds. The one we live in with a physical body, and the one we live in without it. The bridge I saw and bring to you starts when we can direct our brain to step outside the sensory experience. The brain finds it very hard to shut down what it knows and sees every day. It's built to filter our bigger consciousness into a physical experience and to make this illusion look realistic. We trick the brain by telling it that the nonphysical reality is in another room, in another space, and we have to go through an opening, a door that removes the filter on our consciousness and crosses from the sensory experience of our 3-D world to the nonsensory experience of the nonphysical world. To experience this world, we need to mute, or power down, our five senses—sight, hearing, taste, smell, and touch—that keep us grounded in the third dimension. While these senses help our brain navigate this physical experience, they don't serve us well in the nonphysical one. The Temple World enhances our sixth sense, the ability and skill to perceive something or someone that the other senses can't detect. The Temple World is the bridge that heightens the sixth sense and in many ways diminishes the other five.

We Don't Have to Die to Cross Over

While reading about near-death experiences (NDEs), I was caught by the stories of those who'd gone through the experience—they all talked about being greeted by their beloveds and felt a sense of joy and peace. *What if we could experience what they have, only without dying?* I wondered. Others mentioned that they knew time wasn't real and were able to be in different places at once. Many of them talked about being changed when they came back and started to live their lives very differently. The deep sense of connection they felt not only with seeing their beloved but also with being in the space outside of time and marvel at the magnificence of our existence changed them. I was jealous of the peace, compassion, and heightened awareness they brought back with them, their ability to live life more fully, with less fear.

I've never had a near-death experience, and most people I know haven't either. I wanted to find a way to taste what it's like after death without dying, and since reality isn't the way it seems, I initially delved into what scientists refer to as the holographic universe, which proposes that our reality, what we see and experience every day, isn't real. It's a complex hologram, an illusion, alongside the fact that time is also illusionary. The holographic universe supports the idea that our reality is a projection, a grid. Energy. And if it's true that the whole universe is a hologram, then the reality we're experiencing in a linear way is not as it appears. We can't see the grid, the projection, energy, as it really looks. But once we shut down our view here, the bigger reality steps in.

There's an underlying unity beyond the reality we're able to observe and process when we're inside the human body. The hologram, where every part contains the image of the whole, is a beautiful example of this unity. If we do live in a holographic universe, our observation of death as a severing of our connection with our loved ones denies the connection of all things, the wholeness of the cosmos. We're subtracting from that wholeness, which seems to be our tendency. As observers of this 3-D reality, we divide up everything in it and assign labels and values—here, there; come, go; living, dead. We don't see the underlying connection. Yet those who go through NDEs do. In nearly all the stories I've read of people recounting their near-death experiences, when they returned, they brought with them the knowledge of and sense of the unity, the connection, the reality that exists outside time, outside the observation of death.

What if there was a way to experience the connection and wholeness without dying? String theory suggests that microscopic filaments of light connect everyone and everything. What if we could see that? What if we can see the world as it really is? Where everything swims in the same energy and is connected? Where living and nonliving things are not separated? And where we can remove the filter that creates that separation? To make such a world visible, I had to tell the brain that it was visible. I had to tell the brain to look for that reality, to go observe it. When the brain starts to look for the underlying reality we give ourselves a chance at seeing what has been hiding in plain sight.

As I delved farther inside the hidden reality of our existence I began writing more on life after life—the science of it, the evidence for it, the possibility of it. I started telling my readers about the holographic universe, the fact that time isn't real, that we only die in this reality. And if that were true then, what has ended here in our 3-D reality isn't the end. The response was incredible and incredibly heartening to me. My readers were wondering the same things I was. They were excited about this next direction for my work. But, of course, some weren't so happy. In fact, they were furious. They sent emails telling me I was going to hell, where I'd be punished for eternity by God.

I was shocked by the virulence of these responses. But mostly I was surprised that these readers seemed to feel threatened, as if I were trying to take something away from them, rather than add to their understanding of what happens after we die. How could they believe in a God that punishes exploration and curiosity? How could they not believe that there might be other dimensions, realms, worlds we might explore after death, when the heaven they so firmly believe in is itself another realm? With that same wholeness and unity that exists in the deeper reality? We were all believing in the same thing but using different words.

I thought about my childhood and adolescence in Greece. I was raised in a small fishing town. At the beach, in the market, and on the streets God was at the heart of every argument, joke, and deep, meaningful conversation. God was in everything in that town. Every single person I knew believed in God and prayed daily. Greek culture is full of religion and belief in a higher power, and we never considered, let alone discussed, different religions or belief systems to look at this higher power. We believed when you died you went to heaven or to hell. There was nowhere else, or no other words to describe this place we go when we die. Our lives were built on these foundational religious beliefs.

I suspect that my upbringing—at least when it comes to religion—wasn't so different from that of the billions of others who grew up in a similar monotheistic culture, be it Christianity, Islam, or Judaism. Many of my readers have built their lives on similar beliefs. Shaking up these beliefs means shaking up our very upbringing and culture at the same time. This can feel wrong or even frightening. But sometimes we have to shake up the traditional to find, not necessarily the new, but what feels true to who we are now. Reading this book and going through its journey may shake up some of your beliefs. Writing it has certainly shaken some of my own.

When I started researching this book, I believed in a higher power, but I was looking for something I could relate to. I knew it would take a lot for me to believe absolutely that we continue to exist after death in whatever capacity. I wanted to find my own way to a place where I'd have no doubt about the persistence of consciousness, of the persistence of our energy field that connects us to everyone and everything. And I didn't have to die to find out.

While I pull from research about physics and the science of consciousness, and provide data in this book, this book is not here just to teach you how quantum mechanics relates to life—it's also about the experiences you'll have while you shut down your five senses and step out of the 3-D projection to explore a more expansive world, to experience what may happen after we die, and to connect with the people who have. The Temple World exercises will help you see that you're connected to a much larger universe, one that's invisible to the naked eye.

I believe that when we're aware of our limitless, timeless consciousness and our own human powers, we will live our lives from a different perspective, one that includes a life outside the physical boundary that's created by the brain to self-protect. We will believe in our immortal consciousness that is not only eternally present but also action-oriented. In other words, it is a part of the observance and creation of the universe and our existence. We will find the way toward the invisible world and come back from it with tools and experiences that will expand our perspective of life after death, our continued connection with our beloveds, and how our everyday life is created. You see that the path to finding your beloved in the world beyond is also the very same path to your own transcendent state where joy, bliss, and a place where there is no suffering are experienced.

So much of the pain we feel after a loved one dies comes from believing they no longer exist and that we will never see them again. But pain and suffering aren't meant to be part of us forever. We're here to feel joy, not constant grief. What if the person you lost were sitting right there next to you, loving you, but because you're closed to the possibility of other dimensions, you couldn't sense them? Wouldn't that be a shame? I bet someone is sitting right here with me as I'm writing this to you. I hope it's Bjarne, smiling as he reads my computer screen. I hope so because he didn't believe in the continuation of life. Before he died, he told me he was just a wave ready to crash on the shore. That was it. He didn't see the bigger picture—that after crashing, the wave is pulled back into the whole of the ocean, and rises again, crashes again.

As I'm writing this chapter, I can hear him telling me that if he'd known there is no end, he would have spent the last years of his life less afraid. He would have been more present with me and the girls instead of experiencing depression and the fear of death. I wish I could have convinced him about this, but he often tells me that there would have been no way to convince him. He was too strong in his beliefs. Nothing could have changed his mind.

I'm not asking you to change your mind either. All I'm asking is for you to keep an open mind when you read this book, and do the exercises included. So you can experience some of the miracle I have, as have many people in my Temple classes. I want to help you find your beloved so you can carry on living this life fully, knowing that the one you love is somewhere out in the universe living his or her life. This book is here to show you that the most impossible things are possible. A world where grief isn't permanent, the moment of death lasts only a second, and life happens over and over again.

There is no need to be afraid. Welcome to the journey. I can't wait to show you what I've found and help you experience some of it for yourself.

2

the journey begins

I have absolutely no fear of death . . . death is, in my judgment, simply a transition into another kind of reality.

—RAYMOND MOODY

The Temple World is nonlocal; it has no physical location. It's made of pure energy, vibrating at such a high rate that we can't observe it. And the door to that world isn't a physical door, but an opening made, again, of pure energy. While our physical world and the doors in it are also made of energy, that energy is moving much more slowly, which is why it appears solid to our brain. Since our brain is used to seeing a world of edges, curves, and sluggish matter, to begin the trek to deeper understanding of our existence we have to trick it into believing the door to the Temple World is physical. In a sense, we deceive the brain so we can sneak past its limited perception of a 3-D world.

How do you go about tricking your brain? You direct it to perceive the door as something separate from itself, something outside the mind. Something that exists in this reality. The brain can't tell the difference between what's real and what isn't. The moment we tell our brain to look for this door because our eyes are closed, images of that door will appear. In that moment in time, we've given ourselves a gateway to the hidden reality the brain isn't wired to look at. And because our brain operates really well when it labels everything so it can recognize things, I labeled the hidden reality the Temple World.

In this way, we bridge the two worlds and navigate our way from this reality to the one that most have not observed. To the reality of the whole. By labeling the energy. In this case, "Door." You describe the Door—the shape, color, material, defining details—so your brain can believe it's real. Once that happens, the brain opens itself to a bigger experience. This is when your consciousness takes over and sees so much more than that first direction you gave to your brain to see the Door. You start to see the entryway to the Temple World as part of the quantum field. Slowly, as you progress on your journey, your brain stops resisting your new experience of energy.

As we move forward, we need less and less labeling. When we reach what seems to be the edge of the map, the end of this journey, the world we will find ourselves in is a deep experience truly beyond this reality. We will find ourselves consciously inside the quantum field, experiencing it as if we are having a near-death experience, as if we have left our bodies behind and crossed over.

What exactly is the quantum field? In her groundbreaking book *The Field*, journalist Lynne McTaggart writes, "At our most elemental, we are not a chemical reaction but an energetic charge. Human beings and all living beings are a coalescence of energy in a field of energy connected to every other thing in the world. This pulsating energy field is the central energy of our being and our consciousness, the alpha and omega of our existence."[1]

The Temple World is this pulsating energy Lynne McTaggart describes. It's your home away from home. It's seeing the energy with the eyes of the 3-D reality. It is the understanding that the whole also is outside of time and space. Einstein said that time and space are illusions we have created from our imagination. On this journey, we're going to find a way out of those illusions with the creation of the Temple World. Once you find your way out of the illusions and inside the hidden reality by tricking your brain into seeing them as in a physical, geographical location, you start to experience the truth that your brain has been hiding from you so it can survive in this current reality, that this amazing world is nonlocal, always there and always with you. All it is, is a deeper, more hidden world we're unearthing.

In *The Holographic Universe*, Michael Talbot writes, "Our brains mathematically construct objective reality by interpreting frequencies that are ultimately projections from another dimension, a deeper order of existence that is beyond both space and time: The brain is a hologram enfolded in a holographic universe."[2]

It's where we can go to connect to the whole. Connect with the people who are no longer part of this dimension but still are part of the whole universe. The brain filters our beloved out of our experience. And by bypassing the brain filter by labeling the invisible world, I discovered that we can connect and receive information from our loved ones.

The Temple World is what we can finally see when we cease to exist in 3-D reality. It's where our beloveds reside. It's where consciousness is, where matter is, where the whole universe lives, where every galaxy, black hole, and speck of stardust calls home, where we come from, where we go to, and where we are right now even though we don't choose to observe it in this exact moment. Even though the brain stands in the way of experiencing it.

The Temple Journey is a step-by-step journey farther inside this hidden reality, and deeper into the Field. Deeper into the elements that seem invisible to the naked eye.

Why Do We Need to Go on This Journey?

Maybe you're thinking, *I have a church to go to and I haven't had access to the Temple World all of my life, so why do I need this now?* Or maybe you aren't religious and are thinking, *Why go at all?* Because the Temple World is a church you carry within you. It is the divinity that already exists inside of you. It has always been there, but you haven't been aware of it in the way that this journey will allow you to be. It's been this faint knowing that something greater is within you. An awareness of the mystery that surrounds you to which you could never get close enough to understand until you went through a tragedy or a loss and you began to question everything. You asked the question "What is our being here for?" Many times you may have asked, "What is the point of life when all I get is grief and pain? I don't want to do this anymore."

You want to know the answers to some of the biggest questions, such as "Where do we go after we die?" And how is it that our consciousness lives on and on? You'll make your way to the Temple World because the answers you'll get will be for you and only you. These answers will help you connect to an eternal existence of consciousness, allow you the freedom of observing a different reality for yourself while inside your body, and teach you how to let go of your five senses and activate the invisible world that coexists with visible.

It's *your* journey that exists inside the Temple World, not anyone else's. You'll first go there to find solace knowing that death isn't real and that the people you lost are not actually gone forever. Then you'll continue taking the journey because what happens when you're there changes your life here, in this reality. You're not here to suffer and die suffering. You're here to find your way to the truth of your existence. You're here to discover that you have free will. That you've come to learn and grow. Suffering helps us learn, but not when we're stuck and can't find our way to freedom and love again. The Temple World helps you continue on this journey of life.

From the moment you search for the Door until you arrive at the Temple World itself, you'll question what you see, your experience. That's normal. It's a natural part of the process. You are so used to seeing everything with your eyes open. You're so used to seeing the world through this illusion we call the third dimension, so used to using your five senses that asking yourself to let go won't necessarily be easy. And even when you do let go and experience moments of awe, wisdom, love, and peace, you'll question those feelings too. You'll question everything about this journey. It's okay. You're meant to. I did.

One of the reasons I nearly didn't take anyone with me on the Temple Journey was because *I* questioned it. Probably more than anyone else who will read this book. Not only that, but the people in my life with whom I'm close, they questioned this journey, too. They laughed at first. "Really?" they said. "Do you really think this is real? I'm worried about you." And I had to find the courage and strength to trust my own experiences. To trust my sixth sense as much as my other five. I had to find the courage to believe. I'm asking you to do the same. To go forth into the unknown and make it known. To go beyond your wildest dreams and find peace. Because when you do, the experiencing of yourself from another dimension, or/and a place where death doesn't exist, you won't be able to go back to how things used to be.

You'll get to talk to your loved ones every time you visit and the way you feel about your life. You'll find the proof your mind needs to believe so it can create a different future. You'll make dreams come true. Your grief will lighten. You'll take your reentry to life after loss to the next level, one that you couldn't have imagined even before your loss. You will feel happy again, but this time with a level of knowing that surpasses the basic existence of living. The routine of life. The routine of loss. You'll look at yourself not as a passive experiencer but as an active participant. You'll feel content and at peace with who you are. When you come back from each of the journeys, you'll bring with you a real sense of bliss. You'll feel euphoric.

Your relationships with your family and friends will change for the better because you'll feel more loving, accepting, perceptive. You'll feel the connections among all of you. You'll feel less anger and bitterness when recalling past events or current life circumstances because you'll have such a broadened perspective, distance. Your work, projects, everyday tasks will be transformed as you increase your creativity through these experiences inside the Temple World. Since we spend so much of our energy fearing death and doing all we can to avoid it, imagine the freedom you'll feel, the risks you'll take, the dreams you'll pursue if you realize death isn't real. You'll want different things in your life that you never even thought of before or knew you could have. And, of course, you'll have a relationship with the person you lost. You'll experience all these things by learning how to travel to the Temple World and spending time there.

What's the Itinerary?

The Temple Journey consists of five individual journeys that will take you to places you've never consciously visited before. Each of chapters 3 through 7 focuses on one of these journeys. On these journeys, you'll be guided to specific locations, which, in this itinerary, I'll call experiences. Each journey accomplishes two things: it takes you farther from the third dimension, and it helps you to believe and let go.

CHAPTER 3: THE DOOR

The first journey is the Door, which is the entrance to the Temple World. The Door works to encourage the brain to let go of its attachment to its regular 3-D reality, allowing you to move out of your day-to-day reality for the first time. In our daily lives, the brain filters light to make the images we see, and when we turn off the filtering experience, we can perceive what was previously invisible. The very first thing I knew for certain when beginning my own journey is that I could set out on the journey only with my eyes closed, with my five senses reduced. I knew this from my studies of brain science and from my own experience.

The second thing I learned was that the less connected we are to our physical reality, the easier it will be to find the Temple World. From my own experience and those of my students, I discovered that doing things such as floating in the bath, experiencing full-body relaxation during massage, or having our individual energy flow unblocked during acupuncture made the journey significantly easier. To me, these experiences indicate that the Door to the Temple World comes to life when we shut down this 3-D reality. The more real our surrounding world is, the more elusive, absurd, and nonexistent the Temple World seems. On the other hand, the more we let go of the projections our brains create, the more the Temple World comes to life. It's a dance. And we'll learn it.

CHAPTER 4: THE SUPER WATCHER

This journey is perhaps my favorite. After we've crossed through the Door, we meet our Super Watcher for the first time. We all have a guide, a guardian angel, a higher self—it has many names— that lives inside us. It could be another being or our own soul guiding the way. I call it the Super Watcher and on this journey, you get to meet the part of you that has been with you all along from before you can remember.

I call it the Super Watcher because, like any good guide, it is omnipresent and all-observing. It is part of the observer consciousness that created the universe and it is therefore the part of ourselves that helps us to harness our own inherent creativity. Your Super Watcher will be your closest companion on your ride to and through the Temple World—and what a ride it will be. Did you think I was going to let you go there on your own? Not even close. When we connect with the part of ourselves that resides outside this dimension, we find it much easier to connect with our beloved. Consciousness connects with consciousness, instead of a physical body with the ego, what I call the Survivor, and the logical brain. When we let go of the physical body, Survivor, and logical brain, and meet our Super Watcher, it's so much easier to connect with our beloveds.

In the Super Watcher Journey, you'll encounter three primary experiences, which I call the Conversations, the Portal, and the Object.

The Conversations

On all the stops along the way, we get to meet and talk to our loved ones, ask them questions, and see what they've been up to. This is a place of profound healing because we have the opportunity to say all the things we didn't have the chance to say before our loved ones crossed over. I created the Temple Journey for this purpose, but I discovered that this is just one aspect of it. You might experience the meeting of your beloved as soon as you go through the Door; many people do. The Meetings can take place on every journey if you wish for them.

How many Meetings you'll have with your beloved or guide is up to you.

The Portal

Once you've gone through your Door, met your Super Watcher, and had one of your first Meetings with your beloved, you'll ride inside galaxies and faraway worlds. Outside space and time as we typically understand them, beyond this life. You'll enter the Portal and travel among the stars at the speed of light. Our entire universe is made of Portals and black holes that bend space-time. They're shortcuts. Knowing about them and traveling through the Portal on this journey allow our brain to let go even more, losing its concept of time and the need to see things in a linear way.

The Object

One of necessary steps in this journey is finding proof early on for our brains to believe we're in the Temple World. How we observe the Temple World and our experiences there affect our lives in our 3-D reality. The Temple Journey is part of our everyday experience. Throughout the Temple Journey, we'll prove to our brain that it can bring the knowledge, sensations, and experiences it finds in the Temple World back to our 3-D reality. As you can imagine, it's an important exercise.

We look for something within the Temple World that stands out. It could be a necklace, a toy, a set of keys—whatever calls to us. Most of the times it just pops up. We take note of the object in the Temple World, bring it back through the Door during the journey home, and write about it once we're back. In that way we can notice it in our everyday reality. One of the most crucial moments in this process is when you stumble upon your object from the Temple World outside of it, in your regular life. This is when the first deep connection between the two worlds is created. This is when your brain starts to believe in a profound way that what's created inside the Temple World has implications outside it.

CHAPTER 5: THE TEMPLE OF UNIVERSES

On this journey we're introduced to the theory that there are many versions of ourselves—in fact, an infinite number. As part of this learning, we travel to the Temple of Universes. Inside the Temple lies the multiverse, which comprises everything that exists. The whole of space. Time. Matter. Energy. It includes parallel universes—many versions of our lives and of ourselves. When I first found out about the concept of the multiverse, I became fascinated by its implications in our lives. Imagine a world where every version of you is possible. Every step you may have taken, every decision you could have made create new versions of you. Imagine that this experience isn't single but infinite, and you're living only one version. What if you could have access to all of them? I believe that our beloveds, too, exist with us in these other versions.

Inside the Temple of Universes, you experience different probable realities *and* collapse the ones you don't want to observe so they're no longer observable and therefore probable. Don't worry. There is no danger, no reason to be frightened. These universes are simply not what you desire. You're just observing, choosing, and collapsing. You're actively making choices that help your destiny and your lives.

CHAPTER 6: THE TEMPLE MIRROR

I put a mirror inside the Temple of Universes because I wondered what we would witness when we looked at our physical reflection in a nonphysical reality. Can we see ourselves within a nonphysical reality with no limits, no doubts, no worries, no fears? The physical reflection helps journeyers see themselves in the different lives that are possible, have taken place, or are taking place inside the multiverse. Be ready to see yourself in ways that will allow you to expand the perception of yourself. Observe your own magnificence and timeless existence. I'll say no more.

CHAPTER 7: THE FIELD

In the final journey, we experience the quantum field that connects all beings in unity and allows us to heal and to find our purpose. While we're all part of this quantum field that's the very fabric of our existence, we still need to coax our brain into believing it exists. Remember, we don't think we're living our lives inside the Field, even though we are, because we're living inside a very basic 3-D reality. The brain filters out the Field. So to help us understand this phenomenon, we envision a literal field, as in an open space planted with wheat, soy, wild grasses—whatever you see. Directing the brain to go to a specific location makes it much easier to access the Field, until the brain accepts the experience, your consciousness takes over, and it becomes an unbelievable, joyful moment.

Confronting Doubt and Fear

As you make your way on these journeys, your fear center in your brain will become activated and your Survivor self will step in to protect you from experiencing something new. Who is your Survivor? Your Survivor is made of old habits and the resistance triggered by your fear center. The Survivor comprises our automatic thoughts and the concrete physical reality that we're so used to seeing in our lives. It's the part of us that keeps us safe and sidesteps anything that might threaten the safety *it* perceives as important, which means anything that threatens its narrow comfort zone. The Survivor isn't here to keep us from real danger, but imaginary danger, and in doing so, it keeps us from evolution and growth. The Survivor is the part of us that's kept us safe throughout our grief journey. It's the part of us that wants to keep us inside the Waiting Room. The place between the life we left behind after loss and the life we're yet to experience. Inside our safety zone.

As you can imagine, this book is going to give you experiences you may never have had before, and your Survivor is going to try to stop you from having these experiences. It's also going to try to stop you from believing what you are experiencing. It's going to say things such as "This is so ridiculous," or "There's nobody there to reach out to," or even, "Why are you wasting your time with this? The dead are dead forever." The list goes on. Trust me, I've been there, and I still experience my Survivor doubting the magnificence of our world.

The Survivor will do everything it can to stop the Super Watcher from taking you on this journey. It will tell you that you're crazy and this is nonsense. It might even tell you that you're losing your mind and that you need to stop reading this book. It may recruit your family and friends when you start talking about your Super Watcher. They may look at you as though you have three heads. This is when you must trust yourself to know that this journey is real, that this experience you're having isn't just your imagination or your strong need to believe that we don't really die. It's the truth your soul wants you to know in every cell of your body, so you can be free to not only live your life after loss fully, but also to truly expand your awareness of yourself and this life. Knowing that your Super Watcher travels with you everywhere you go and never dies is key to the success of your journey.

Your Survivor isn't all bad. It's a big part of our physical world after loss. It wants to keep you away from anything that makes you afraid or involves a new beginning or change. The Survivor wants to keep things in the status quo. It wants to keep you from risking losing anything more than what you've already lost. Sometimes the Survivor is going to be very difficult to quiet. But I've helped thousands of people send their Survivors away. The good news is that we *can* get a break from it. The bad news is that it will always come back. But you can become really good at extending the Survivor's vacation time.

One of the ways in which you can stop the Survivor from reacting to the perceived threat that's taking place will be to immerse yourself in communities of people who want to experience the same journey as you do—people who want to explore the non-physical world. We have a group on Facebook called Where Did

You Go? You can search for it. Or you can create your own Temple Circle. Without creating a tribe of like-minded individuals who are on this same journey, your Super Watcher will need to work overtime to keep focused on new probabilities.

You don't have to join a group, but it's better to read this book with at least one other person. This will help validate the Temple Journey for you and allow for an extraordinary experience. In many ways, the Temple Journeys need to be acknowledged and validated by others. For them to feel real, they need to be felt and heard. The more of us who experience the journeys together, the more we can help others do the same, and by doing so, many more people will be able to bridge this gap between the physical reality and the nonphysical one.

The Collective Journey

The Temple Journey is ultimately an individual journey. One you take on your own with the whole universe by your side. But it can be enhanced by the validation and the sharing that take place within a group. If you choose to take this journey as part of the collective, then gather a group together. This group can be a group of two, ten, or as many as you want. You can connect with like-minded people on my Star Letters, Second Firsts sites, or my Facebook pages (you'll find links to these pages and, as I said earlier, a private Facebook group in the Resources section at the back of this book). Or you could find members for your group in your local church, in your neighborhood, or perhaps your whole family can read this book together. The exercises in the book work wonderfully for children. Imagine what their life would be like if your children could access the Temple Journey early in their life.

As you gather your group and ask that they read this book and work the exercises with you, share with them exactly what the Temple Journey is about, and let them know your beliefs about the persistence of consciousness. Connecting with your group on these issues is crucial. They, too, have to believe there's something else out there. Something real that we can't see.

Meet once a week, either on Skype, Facebook, or in person to go through each chapter together. Make sure you do all the exercises, because each of them builds on the one before to construct a bridge from the physical world to the nonphysical world.

While working *through* this book with a group is important, creating a community of like-minded individuals is important *after* you finish reading as well. (You can continue to meet with the group you've worked with, or work with a new one. Again, see the Resources section to help you connect with others who are on this journey.) Why? Even though the Super Watcher is totally on board with this new way of looking at our lives, the people around us may not be.

Sound Vibrations for Every Journey

I've created a Temple World sound vibration to accompany each of the individual journeys. These sound vibrations enhance the brain's ability to release its hold on the present reality more easily and set out more quickly on each journey. They also, critically, help to block as much sensory input as possible during each journey. These two benefits combined create a meditation-like state.

BINAURAL BEATS

I have been fascinated with binaural beats for a while now, and I had to include them in this journey. "Binaural beats" is a confusing term because it seems like a phrase describing an external sound—a type of beat. But a binaural beat is actually a type of brain response—a shift in brain activity—that happens when we hear two different frequencies at the same time. The brain responds to the difference between the two frequencies by hearing an imaginary third frequency. That third frequency creates an effect, an experience. Some of the effects are better sleep, relaxation, physical healing, and reduction of stress and anxiety. Having a relaxed brain while journeying to the Temple World is crucial.

DRUMS

I asked Jeff Suburu, the musician who worked with me to create the Temple Journey sound vibrations, to weave drumbeats throughout. He sent about six samples of drumbeats, and I kept sending each one back until we found the right one. Why? Because the beat of a drum can bring forth a trance state. According to scientist Melinda Maxfield, PhD, when listening to consistent drumbeats, our brains shift to a low theta brain wave state and become more experiential, more dreamlike. She writes about the drumming and chanting that take place in shaman and Hindu healer circles and how they induce specific brainwave states for transcending consciousness.[3]

For each journey you take, you can listen to the sound vibrations of the Temple World, your own music, or nothing at all. Even though the vibrations enhance the journeys, you'll discover that the Temple World does come through regardless of whether you use these sounds. But using the vibrations will help you take a deeper journey. To download the Temple Journey sound vibrations, go to the Resources section to find the link, and then before you take the journey each day, play the appropriate sound vibration on your playlist if that's what you choose to listen to. You can download the vibrations on your phone or computer.

What You Need to Bring with You

Remember to have something on hand—a notebook, an iPad, etc.—to record your experience after the journey. During the journey experience you will not be typing or writing anything. But once you are back here, I would advise you to write about what you saw and felt. You will also need to find pictures online that match all the things you observed while in the Temple World. You may also want an electronic device to play the optional sound vibration that accompanies the exercises. It could be your phone, your iPod, or your computer—the sounds are easily downloadable.

Conclusion

We need a strong sense of self, because self-observation is key to this path. We're going to be challenged, and observation is critical to the process of change. We no longer want to respond to the world around us without conscious thought and focused attention. Imagine seeing your life from a place of true knowing and not from one of automatic survival. It will feel as though you installed a pause between you and your life. You'll feel as if you can make time stop long enough for you to think, decide, and just simply know what you should do. We need to regulate our neocortical regions so we can increase the regulation of our feelings. These regions have to do with our sensory perception, generation of motor commands, spatial reasoning, conscious thought, and, language. We'll be creating new pathways. New brain maps. These brain maps will allow for a belief in a bigger and vaster world, one that includes those you've lost.

As we create new beliefs and thus new realities, we have to be very aware about how far off these new beliefs are from our old ones. If they're too far off, our brain will simply reject them and deny them. This is the reason why the Temple Journey is made of steps and experiences, so you can slowly move further and further inside the Temple World. We need to step slowly into our right hemisphere—the more imaginative, creative hemisphere—more often to challenge the status quo. We need to be less logical, less black and white, so we can revise our view of the world. And if you need to read and experience this book more slowly, then you must do just that. Maybe even a chapter every two weeks, rather than one.

I'm going to be daring you to continually expand the edge of your reality with each chapter. You have the ability and the knowledge to do this. I want you to remember that what you see with your eyes is not all there is. As a matter of fact, it's very little of what's out there. I have this force inside me that pushes me every day to help you see the magnificence of the world that surrounds you, a world that includes the person you lost. And no, I don't have all the answers and never will. But you'll get to experience so much more than you thought was possible. This is not a magic carpet ride. It's a ride that everyone deserves to be on. And it's real. Get ready for surprises *and* to be doubted by your friends. Be okay with that. This is your journey, not theirs. Here we go. You, me, and everyone here—let's do this.

3

the door

Reality is merely an illusion, albeit a very persistent one.

—ALBERT EINSTEIN

A re you saying I'll see my Annie again?"

I'd just received an email from Joan about registering for the Temple class. Her daughter, who was eighteen, had been killed three years earlier by a drunk driver.

"I have always believed she's still alive," Joan wrote, "just not the way we are."

Joan had dreamed of Annie only three times since she'd passed away. Those dreams left Joan filled with joy, and she wanted more. "I wish every day to find a way to be with her," Joan wrote. "Don't worry, I'm not saying I want to die or anything like that, even though that crossed my mind in the beginning, but if there's a way to get to Annie, I want to know what that is."

"There are no guarantees, of course," I told her, "and everyone's journey through the Door is different."

"I don't care about guarantees," she answered. "I care about having a chance."

And with this declaration, Joan's Temple Journey began.

When our class met for the first time and completed the Door Journey, Joan shared her experience.

"My feet felt light, as though I were suspended in midair. I was moving forward, even though I was surrounded by darkness and had no idea where I was going. I couldn't see a thing. No Door that you instructed us to look for. Nothing. I started to panic. Where was my Door? What if I couldn't find it? What if I couldn't get through to see Annie? Then suddenly, my thoughts still swirling, I saw not an open Door, but an opening that widened into the darkness, with light piercing through. How could I really trust this? I thought, then, *but what if she's there waiting for me?* I was scared. I felt unsafe, even though I knew I was still sitting on my chair. But I wanted to dare and do this for her. For myself. Suddenly, superfast, I was through the opening—I felt vibrations on my body from the opening, but I went through so fast, that's all that registered. Then I found myself in the middle of a field. I was spinning, as though I had vertigo. As though I was physically moving somewhere else, away from here.

"In the midst of the spinning, I felt Annie's presence. It's hard to explain. I couldn't see her quite yet, but I could feel her. A profound feeling of peace replaced my fear. It was as if she knew I was there and was waiting for me. I'm crying during the spinning, during the knowing of her being there. It's overwhelming. I've missed her so much.

"Then the spinning stopped. She was closer. I knew she wasn't the only one there. I felt others. But I was focused only on her. I felt so much peace here, where she was. Where everyone was. No one spoke. This seemed to be a place without words. And for me, without heartache. I wanted to stay there forever. Then, just like that, while I was immersed in this unspoken world, I saw her. She looked so happy, the way she had when she was about to go out with her friends for the evening. She was wearing her blue jeans and her favorite turtleneck blouse her sister bought for her for her birthday that year. It was as if she were coming through the way she did when she was the happiest.

"I could hear your voice, Christina, guiding me back, but I didn't want to leave. It felt like home and Annie was there. Why would I want to leave? I felt a huge surge of sadness and fear in going back through the opening. I wanted to stay with Annie and this amazing sense of love, light, and energy that was surrounding me. But I knew I had to come back

"Was I just *imagining* this? Joan looked straight at me. The expression on her face told me she was questioning everything about the journey.

"If I was sitting in this chair," Joan said, "and Annie's been gone three years, then how did we meet? How did it feel like I saw her, but there was something different about her? It was her, but it wasn't her. She felt wise, calm. Going through the opening filled me with a sense of joy I haven't felt in a while, if ever, definitely not since her passing. I still feel the joy and peace from that world on the other side of the door, and from being with Annie, from knowing she's happy." Joan wiped tears from her cheeks. "Will it stay, this feeling? I want it to stay. I can be happy again if this, whatever *this* is, stays with me somehow."

I told her it can but it doesn't always. But as she continues the

Temple World Journey, each time she comes back from that world and opens her eyes in this one, she'll bring a little more of that world back with her. I tried not to say too much, just enough for her to get an idea of how the journey will unfold. I want her to have her own experience.

Joan looked relieved when I told her she might bring the feeling back.

I could see that she had a new sense of knowing that wasn't there before—as though something had changed in her perception of life after death, her understanding of what happened to her daughter.

What Will You Experience?

The goal of the Door Journey is to bring back with us what we can—as Joan hoped to bring back the emotions of her experience—to elevate *this* life. To move away from the ego, from fear, and from the limited perspective of consciousness and human life that we have lived in thus far.

While you may share similarities with others, your journey will be as unique as your fingerprints, your DNA, and the way you look. When we begin the Door Journey, you'll experience a sense of anticipation and uncertainty, and because of this, you and I will take this journey slowly and with a sense of adventure and awe, being open to seeing whatever appears, without trying to create or imagine it, and without rejecting it. Just be with it.

The Door has energy. Just as you do. It's made of the same stuff you're made of. Going through the Door, some of you may experience spinning, as Joan and a few others in the class who went on the Door Journey did.

The purpose of the Door Journey is to help you understand that there's a gateway inside your house, your bedroom, your office, your backyard—wherever you sit down to take this journey. Wherever you are, the Door is there. You don't have to die to experience crossing through. You don't have to say a special prayer, or even be asleep. Even the beautiful sounds that have been created and recorded specifically for this journey are there to help you step into the part of you that remembers the place beyond the Door, or gateway.

You'll be guided to walk slowly toward what you can see as a Door, or opening, with your eyes closed. You may feel a bit disoriented, which is your brain's response to the newness of the experience. It will pass. You will be asked to trust your own experience and to feel safe doing so. You're safe in this reality where your body lives and experiences life. You're going to ask your brain to take you as far as it can, and then, as you go through the Door, let go of the logical, linear, and spatial physical experience of the body and switch to letting your consciousness guide you.

I attribute the spinning that Joan and a few of the other members of the class went through to that switch. Once you're through the Door, your brain most likely won't try to stop your experience for at least a few seconds. But if it does and you are back in the chair, try to take a deep breath and slowly start the journey again. Once you are through and able to stay you'll be seeing and feeling this new place more clearly and intensely than you expected. And even though this first step isn't meant for the actual meeting of your loved one to take place, for some people it does. But from my point of view, this first step is for you to experience the difference in vibration, energy, feeling, and being. It's to prepare you for the bigger journey to connect with your beloved. Your person. The love or loves of your life.

To me, it has always been so very surprising when I see people meeting their beloveds as soon as they go through the opening. While I'm no longer surprised at these meetings, I was at first. I had not anticipated the immediate connection and meetings taking place. But there they were. Immediate. Unforgettable. And real.

What will you experience? A shift. A moment or two of discomfort. An experience of the invisible world you're immersed in. It is you who gets to visit your beloved, not the other way around. You get to go and find them this time. And they're grateful that you are. This is your visitation, not theirs. This is you seeking them out.

I know now how happy these visits have made those who've passed. I know because they didn't even wait for me to guide people beyond the threshold. They were right there, and according to those who took the Door Journey, full of joy and in complete bliss.

Why a Door?

After my husband died, and I searched for him everywhere, I felt like I had hit a wall. I could not connect with him. I could not find him. There were not only impossible physical obstacles to overcome, but also obstacles inside my beliefs and thoughts. I felt that even if he were somewhere else, that place was far away from me. But then I came to learn that this reality of ours is not what it seems. We are energy, not matter. Three-dimensional reality is an illusion. A field of energy is the only truth. A truth that is so hard to accept from the perspective of the physical dimension. But one that is infinite and timeless. One that has the people we lost inside of it. And if you want, it can be a place you can visit, too.

The reality you're experiencing right now, holding this book, is a projection your mind is using to help you understand this earthly experience. The loss of your beloved is also not real beyond this reality. The Temple World is where we came from and where we get to go once we're not in this body. The thing is, we don't have to die to find out that death isn't real. And we don't have to die to meet the people we lost again.

In developing my first Temple Journey class, I knew I needed a way to help my students get to that other reality where they could visit their loved ones easily. I needed to find a way to help their brains accept the experience from the get-go. The very first question I asked myself when creating this initial journey of crossing over was, how can someone go to that other reality easily, every day, without having to struggle with the boundaries the brain has created?

There are so many constraints that exist in this reality. Though these constraints are uncomfortable, they give this world structure, and structure feels safe. We believe it's comfortable. But in truth, there isn't anything comfortable about being stuck inside a set of rules and laws with no control or ability to move into a dimension of potentiality that is our birthright. But to find a way out of this reality, we have to play by its rules—the rules of the brain.

The brain takes its job very seriously, and it does it extremely efficiently—too efficiently, if you ask me. The brain's role is to take the information given to it and process that information. The brain searches for patterns and predictability in organizing that information, which makes our reality more comprehensible, more neatly organized. Our brain trains us to revisit those patterns. For example, most of our days are exactly the same because we've created a routine: an experience that keeps us safe through predictability. We grab a cup of coffee every morning. We go to work at the same time. We take the same route home. Predictability means we don't have to think much, create much, or be in a new way. We just go through an automatic cycle that the brain loves.

I talk a lot about our brain's love of patterns in my Life Reentry work. I explain how when tragedy or loss causes us to exit the routines of our everyday lives, our brain takes us to a place I call the Waiting Room. The part of our brain that tries so very hard to keep us inside the Waiting Room, inside the known, the familiar, and routine, I've named the Survivor (the fear center inside our brain). As I mentioned in the last chapter, the Survivor tries very hard to keep us not only inside what we have always known, but in the case of the journey we'll take in this book, also inside this 3-D world that operates in a linear, predictable way.

The loss of routine can feel like a threat to the brain. The Waiting Room is a "safe" place, where because of inertia you do nothing and are therefore out of what the brain perceives as harm's way. The Waiting Room is the place between two lives: the life we left behind because of the loss, and the life we can have if we find a way out. But it's very hard to find a way out, because the brain doesn't like change. So the Survivor leads your life after loss. The Survivor will do everything it can to convince you that whatever you're trying to do in the Temple World isn't real and isn't good for you.

Change is a challenge to patterns and predictability. Whether we're leaving the Waiting Room or going through the Door to the Temple World, we have to sneak out of familiar terrain to the unfamiliar by giving our brain predictability. The brain is lazy, to say it simply and directly. And since we're taking a massive leap toward a new state of consciousness, we need a familiar transitional image to reduce the fear response of the brain. That's where the Door comes in. The Door creates an opening that allows you to enter into another dimension safely and without having to experience a near-death experience, an out-of-body experience, or even sit in deep meditation.

Working *with* the Brain

In his book *Biocentrism*, Robert Lanza quotes an old Zen saying, "Name the colors, blind the eye" to illustrate that the "intellect's habitual ways of branding and labeling creates a terrible experiential loss by displacing the vibrant, living reality with a steady stream of labels."[1] In other words, when we are in our thinking mind, we close ourselves to the expansive possibilities available to us. For example, we might use one word, "blue," to describe a thousand different shades. And yet that word helps us to make sense of our reality. It's the same with the Door. We need a way for our brain to initially comprehend and accept a challenging idea—that there is a reality beyond this one.

By using a familiar symbol and label—"Door"—we are working *with* the brain to provide it with a sense of security, so we can actually open ourselves to a new experience, a new way of understanding. The Door signifies an entryway to an experience outside of our reality. Seeing the Door gives your brain permission to leave behind this solid reality and enter another form of existence, which I call the potentiality state, where you can realize your potentials: all possible outcomes for past, present, and future. It also exists without the need of our five senses. As a matter of fact, the more unaware of our senses we are, the faster we can experience this entryway into the dimension of potentiality. The Door leads us to our natural state, which is the state we were in when we were without a body. We have come from a nonphysical dimension, and once we go through the Door, we go back to that nonphysical state. We're not completely disconnected from our consciousness while we're in a physical body.

Most likely, the last time you truly were outside this 3-D reality was when you were a baby, connected with the all, your body not separate from the space around you. But over time, your parents taught you that you're an individual, that everything outside your physical body—your mom, your sibling, the swing in your backyard—was something other than you. They also taught you about your body, your language, and the idea of possession, that your books and toys belonged to you and that you were responsible for taking care of them. Essentially, all these lessons served to strengthen the ego, whose job is to keep your body safe and protected. They taught you these concepts so you could survive in this reality.

Now this book comes along questioning some of the things you were taught by the people who loved you. We have to be gentle with this experience because if we treat the brain as our friend who is taking the Door Journey alongside us (at first, anyway, until it becomes used to the Temple World and lets our consciousness take over), this important journey will be easier. The brain is needed to get us into and out of that experience. After all, we choose this reality for now. The ability to enter and exit the Temple World stems from the skill of being able to bring our brain along with us and let it go at the right time. We work with our brain, not against it. One of the things I learned over the years was that we love our Survivor the most, because of its protective mechanism. It's the part of us that's kept us breathing and living after loss. But we must also learn to let it go when we venture out, and, in the case of the Temple World, beyond what we have known before.

We want to take the brain with us on the journey without any rebellion. We want to go forth whole and multidimensional, without leaving behind our psychology, our concepts, and our social nature. We want to bring them all with us. They're part of who we are. Our brain needs these aspects of ourselves to help us make sense of the Temple Journey.

The Door is, I believe, the very first step toward finding our way to a reality that includes nonphysicality, limitless possibilities, and a sense of creation beyond the boundaries of what we are accustomed to, where the consciousness of the people we have lost still exists.

Our mind and soul have access to many realities beyond this one. The Door Journey helps open the door to those realities. And to do so, we need the cooperation of our brain and our body, even as we necessarily "let go" of them while we are in the Temple World. But that letting go is, of course, only temporary. We must and should return to our 3-D reality, bringing back with us what we can to live this life more fully. We are more than just this body and this basic way of operating through our 3-D system. When we go beyond this reality, we find our way outside of loss and pain. We cannot and should not stay there, but we should allow the experience to alleviate the pain, alienation, and sorrow we all carry with us. And we need the brain to cooperate in doing just this.

We must really find a way to see beyond the illusion and then find a way to step outside the predictable patterns we live in, to change the brain so it can create what we want it to create. It's a long way to go, especially when what you're perceiving looks nothing like the solidity of your kitchen table. You can't aim and shoot. You have to close your eyes. And that is no easy task for a mind that looks for solid targets and surefire routes to reach them.

The Door will help your mind aim at something specific, something solid, something it can understand instead of aiming at nothing, in the empty space of nowhere. Because that's how the brain understands a place without matter—it thinks it is empty. But we are going to a place where there are fewer rules; no time; and above all, no death.

Just as with time, death isn't real. Just as with time, this solid formation—this book—you see in front of you isn't real. This reality is a creation of our mind where we live in a linear setting for some seventy-nine years, and then we die. We're going to try to use the Door to start a slow exit from this belief—that we die. It's going to be a slow exit, because a fast exit won't work. A fast exit will only create more doubts, more fear, and more clinging to this reality we perceive with our five senses.

> You exist in time, but you belong to eternity. You are a penetration of eternity into the world of time. You are deathless, living in a body of death. Your consciousness knows no death, no birth. It is only your body that is born and dies.
>
> —OSHO

Where Are You Going?

Though the Door Journey is not a meditation, I believe it takes us to a state similar to that achieved in meditation. According to Bernard Haisch, Peter Russell, author of *The Global Brain* and faculty member at the Institute of Noetic Sciences, describes that state this way: "In everyday life we all experience three states of consciousness: the awake state, in which we experience awareness

and the objects of our consciousness originate in the physical reality around us; the dream state, in which we experience awareness,
but the objects of our consciousness have some internal origin;
and the deep sleep state, in which there is no awareness. The state
achieved in meditation is a fourth distinct state, in which there is
awareness, indeed profound awareness, but awareness of nothing
but consciousness itself."[2]

Similarly, the Door Journey takes you to the threshold of the
Temple World, a place that is pure consciousness, or put another
way, the world you're from and go to when this reality is no longer part of your consciousness. When you die you only die in the
reality your consciousness has created to experience the physical
world. In other words, when we meet with death here we are
met with awareness and knowing that belong and have always belonged to us. When your loved one died in this reality, he or she
did not die in the reality of their awareness and their consciousness. The only way you can reach them seems to be when you get
to step out of this physical reality and inside your own awareness
of the field of consciousness that we all reside in. Near-death experiences consist of moments when we're able to leave this physical
reality our consciousness has created and jump into the awareness
of consciousness; timelessness; joy; and, above all, immortality.
Where is all this? Inside your consciousness.

The Door is taking you inside. Yes, inside. Yourself. If you
could only see the vastness of reality that lives within you and
outside this solid illusion of our world, you'd be blown away. The
seemingly outside world is inside your mind, so the world inside
is also the world outside. They are one and the same, separate

only in our 3-D reality. Since our brain needs these delineations to navigate and comprehend our world, I'm referencing inside and outside to help explain what your brain needs to get to this place outside of space and time. Inside us live the whole universe in all its dimensions, and last but not least, the people we've lost.

During that first class, when people came back from their first Door Journey and shared their experiences with the group, it was as if they'd all had a near-death experience. They marveled at the bliss and joy they felt when they crossed over. And even though this first journey is about crossing and coming back—nothing more—surprisingly, many people saw their beloveds. It was as if their beloveds were waiting for *their* loved ones on the other side. How could that be? How could they be somewhere else, yet we could get to them in the blink of an eye? How could they be gone from our world, yet we could just drop in for a visit?

As I mentioned earlier, our ability to switch off this 3-D reality by focusing on the Door and to turn our attention to the invisible energy, dimensions, and the holographic universe allows us to see, hear, and experience our beloveds. It's immediate. They have always been here, there, and everywhere. We just haven't been open to them. When we were, it was much more immediate than I ever expected. I thought the brain would hold on to us much longer than it does, and we would hold on to it even longer still. However, this is but a journey home, where our loved ones have gone to wait for us. We're looking for and going through a Door entrance outside time and space, outside the linear understanding of our lives. When we step outside of time, we also step outside of death and enter eternity.

In Biocentrism, Robert Lanza writes, "If one could travel at lightspeed, one would find oneself everywhere in the universe at once."[3] I felt so excited reading that. While our physical body might not be able to travel at light speed on its own, I believe our consciousness can, that outside this 3-D reality we can be everywhere at once. If that's so, if we can be outside time and space with everyone we've lost, then death isn't real. If we could revisit the people who were once with us in this life, then death is only a temporary experience. A made-up experience.

I read on and got goose bumps. "Because time doesn't exist, there is no after death. Except the death of your physical body in someone else's now. . . . It's simply impossible to go anywhere. You will always be alive. . . . At death, we finally reach the imagined borders of ourselves."[4]

In short, we die in someone else's reality, not in our own.

Bjarne, my husband, died. But he died only in my reality. He didn't die in his. His reality continued in a different way, outside of the 3-D world and away from the limitations of his body. I will never be certain about his exact location because he's everywhere always. Time only exists here.

We have assumed this reality. We have assumed that consciousness is inside the body. We've also assumed that when this reality ends, because our bodies shut down, we cease to exist. And this is partially true. In the way we perceive the world—translating light and magnetic fields into color and sound through our brains and bodies—we cease to exist. But when this body ages and dies and we're without our eyes, our legs, our ears, we'll still *be*, just not in the way we used to. We'll be processing the universe in a different way.

We only die in someone else's reality, not in ours. Thank you, Robert Lanza, for putting into words what others couldn't. When I read his explanation of how death doesn't exist, I felt like I got back all the people I had loved and lost. Including Bjarne. He is dead for me but not for him. He only died in my reality. And that to me is everything.

> What do I think happens when we die? I think we enter into another stage of existence or another state of consciousness that is so extraordinarily different from the reality we have here in the physical world that the language we have is not yet adequate to describe this other state of existence or consciousness. Based on what I have heard from thousands of people, we enter into a realm of joy, light, peace, and love in which we discover that the process of knowledge does not stop when we die. Instead, the process of learning and development goes on for eternity.[5]
>
> —RAYMOND MOODY, PARANORMAL:
> MY LIFE IN PURSUIT OF THE AFTERLIFE

Survivor-Free Zone

It's okay to doubt the power of the Door. I know that it may be hard to believe that an entry that seems a fabrication of our mind can open an entryway to feelings and experiences beyond the limits of our daily life. That this Door will really take us to a place where we can meet our loved ones again. Where we can create a life beyond our wildest expectations. Of course we doubt. We're human, after all. We're meant to see everything in a physical form, inside a 3-D reality.

But how do you go to the place beyond this solid, 3-D reality while perhaps struggling with doubt? How do you venture to a place you can't experience with your five senses, where you're gently required to find your sixth? How do you go beyond the fake walls our brains construct that feel so real to us? Not everyone finds it easy to transcend this very solid physical reality. We do it every day in our dreams, however—dreams about flying, dreams that are visits from your beloved. I know, too, that many people, perhaps most, have had experiences that can't be explained within the rules of this 3-D reality.

One of the first things I ask students before the Temple class even begins is, "What signs from the world beyond have you experienced so far?" Everyone I've talked with has had a sign or an experience they couldn't explain. These experiences are always breathtaking. Some people have awakened in the middle of the night and seen their beloved standing at the foot of their bed. Even though, at the time, this experience was very real (and, yes, sometimes frightening), they woke up the next morning questioning themselves, as I did when it happened to me. Yet these unexplainable experiences help open you to the possibility of a Door.

If you feel you haven't had a sign or an experience that's out of the ordinary, go back to moments where you dismissed something you felt, saw, or thought about. That dismissal is the Survivor trying to keep you in a world that's logical, safe, and familiar. When you go back to that moment, question the Survivor that dismissed it, and ask yourself, *What if what I saw or experienced or thought I saw or experienced was really there?* I know you've experienced moments of not knowing what something is, and I also know that you, too, can go to the other side of the Door and find yourself somewhere else. How am I so certain about these points? Because you and I have come from the same place, have been created in the same way, and are made to access worlds beyond this one. You already have the ability and the tools to go through the Door. You just need to prove it to yourself. To remember.

The Door Journey

The Door Journey, the first in the Temple Journey, allows you to see a reality that's not filtered through your brain, but instead experienced directly by your consciousness. This journey is the first step in developing the belief, the *knowing*, that your beloved only died in this reality and not in the bigger consciousness experience.

There are two main parts in this journey—seeing the Door and crossing through it. Both will help you understand that you create your reality and that death is not real. Remember, our consciousness is the creator of physical matter, and the truth about our existence goes beyond materialism, chemistry, and biology.

The Door Journey can take place daily, if you feel up to it. I hope you will. In the beginning of this new experience, daily practice is incredibly helpful. Every time you go through the Door, feel the energy and allow yourself to expand and truly step into this new space. There are wisdom and certainty there. There is knowing. There is truth. Be open to what you experience. Notice what's changing in your life by just going beyond the Door, in this new place your consciousness created.

What you'll get to experience will shatter some of the doubts we all have. I've seen this happen so often, so I truly believe that you, too, will experience these huge shifts. As I've said, part of this journey requires proof, and we'll find it. And that's why I'm going to be looking for proof, and why we're going to be looking for your stories after you've done this. The more you share your experience in this world, the more real it will be.

Find a comfortable chair in a quiet place where you won't be disturbed. Read the instructions below once or twice before you close your eyes to take the journey. Remember to have something on hand—a notebook, an iPad, etc.—to record your experience after the journey. If you'd like, you can play the corresponding sound vibration (see Resources) or other music, or simply proceed in silence. Relax your shoulders. You're in a safe space.

1. Close your eyes and, gently and slowly, imagine taking steps toward a Door. At first the Door might seem far away, but see yourself approaching it slowly. It might even help to look at your feet as you are walking, and then slowly look up (of course with your eyes closed). When you first see your Door, take a good look at it; notice the details. This Door is breathtaking in every way. This Door is part of you and it is unique to you. It's always been there, waiting for you.

2. Now, start approaching the Door. As you approach, wisdom and light emanate from the Door. Feel yourself absorbing this

light, this wisdom. The Door can be open or closed. It can have a handle or not. It might even be a simple opening instead of a traditional entrance.

3. Take a few more steps, drawing closer and closer to the Door. Gently walk through the Door. As you do so, you experience energy, joy, bliss—feelings deeper and more wonderful than you can imagine.

4. Once you cross the threshold, look around you. You are in the entryway to the Temple World. How big is it? How small is it? Is there a place to sit? Is it circular? Is it narrow? Is it vast? When you look around you, what stands out? How does it feel to be there? You are here not only to witness, not only to see, but also to feel everything that this place is about.

5. Now find a place to sit down, if you wish, or you can continue walking. You feel a sense of calm and certainty and knowing.

6. Take as much time as you need to absorb this reality—how it looks, how it feels. Is there anyone there? What are you seeing or feeling? Be open to whatever comes to you. If you see your beloved, take your time having this experience with them. If you don't, that is okay. You are just meant to experience the crossing in this first step inside the Temple World. Take in the shift in vibration and energy. Listen to the sounds from the recording. Make sure you capture what you see in your heart and your mind and slowly turn back toward the Door.

With a deep breath, cross its threshold back to everyday reality. Slowly come back in this world, to your chair, and when you're ready, open your eyes.

7. Take a deep breath and sit quietly, letting your body integrate back into your everyday reality. Notice how you feel different. When you are ready, get out your notebook or device and make a few notes—you'll want them later. Feel the peace that remains and know that you can make the journey through the Door anytime you want. If you belong to a group, make sure you share your experience with them as soon as you can.

Your Homework for this Week

You've just completed the first journey within the Temple World. You're probably still feeling a little new to all this and it's important that you share this journey with someone else. Since much of this journey requires visualizing, observing, and inner seeing, validation of this experience is important. Our goal is to bring the journey from the inside to the outside. The more we can reflect on it and talk about it, the more your Door and your crossing can come to life. Also, look for your Door in your external world. My guess is that you'll find it. Most of my class participants went online to a site like Pinterest to find an image of their Door, or something as close to it as possible. Some even said they found the Door in their neighborhood or even another town they visited that week. Then they all shared their image of the Door in their online group.

As I said, it is a good idea to take this journey through the Door every day for at least a week. You do not need to rush to go to the next journey. If you feel you're ready to move to the next chapter, do so. Trust yourself in this process.

I have now taken many walks through the Door, and the Door changes over time, as does what you see on the other side. The journeys are never the same. Every time you go through the Door it will feel more familiar, and you'll experience and see new things. Witness them. Share them. Remember them. For example, notice your stride—how it changes when you go to the Temple World, and how that change is reflected in your 3-D reality. For me, this change was a surprise. My walk in this reality started to mimic my stride to the Door. With each journey, my walk to the Door became increasingly stronger and more fearless, as did my walk in this 3-D world.

You've just embarked on a new journey, one that you never thought was possible. You stepped inside a new reality, one that was invisible to you but has always been there. Embarking on this journey, you were open to finding your way to your beloved against all odds, against the obstacles thrown at you by the laws of this physical reality and the automatic pathways of your brain. Congratulations on being courageous and saying yes to this unexpected journey. Now buckle up for what's to come next. I know it will shatter the illusion of the third dimension even more, and it will get you closer to and more familiar with the person you love and have actually not lost.

4

the super
watcher

We are a way for the universe to know itself.
Some part of our being knows this is where we came from.
We long to return. And we can, because the cosmos is
also within us. We are made of star stuff.

—CARL SAGAN

I don't know how it's possible, Christina, but when I heard you say, 'Allow your Super Watcher to travel outside of you,' I saw an orb of light coming from my body," Denise said during our class Skype call. We'd just finished the group Super Watcher Journey, where we travel through a Portal beyond the Door. She stared off to the side, perplexed. "I don't think I'll be able to see or feel anything since I haven't even dreamed about him yet."

Denise lost her husband, Dave, two months earlier from lung cancer, and she was feeling numb from her grief. She'd mentioned many times how she hadn't been able to cry yet.

"So your Super Watcher looked like an orb?" I reflected back to her.

"It did. I thought, from the descriptions in class, that my Super Watcher would look more like me. I wasn't expecting an orb."

I smiled. "Denise, this is the beauty of the work we're doing here, we don't know what we're going to encounter as we travel farther into the Temple World. It's not your brain that's creating the experience; it's your consciousness connecting with another realm. I paused. "Did you see Dave while there?"

"I saw him but very faintly. I questioned if I was really seeing him or I was creating him there," she said. "At first I saw him from the corner of my eye, or it felt like the corner of my eye, standing much farther away, kind of off to the side, just watching me. Then he came with us inside the Portal without saying anything. I must admit, I was so taken when we entered the Portal that I sort of lost track of him. I didn't look for him as much. Isn't that strange?"

I sensed a little bit of guilt in her words. "Not strange at all, Denise. This realm brings forth an experience that is so beautiful that sometimes it can take us away from our grief and longing. What did you find on the other side of the Portal?" I asked.

"At first I couldn't find anything." I had asked the class to look for an object on this journey—the Super Watcher Journey. "It was as if there was nothing there for me to find. But I walked around a little bit and soon saw Dave sitting at a table. There was a necklace on the table in front of him and off to the side. I walked toward him, and the closer I got, the more he smiled, as though to indicate I was going in the right direction. I picked up the necklace. It had a pendant with three blue stones. I've never seen a necklace like that before." Denise thought for a moment. "I picked up the necklace and looked at Dave again. He was smiling, watching as I clasped it around my neck."

"How did that feel?"

"I was expecting to feel guilty about taking the necklace from this world to one he was no longer part of, but I didn't. Seeing Dave smiling at me, feeling this deep contentment emanating from him, I felt happy. I knew how he felt by just being next to him, I don't know how, but I did," Denise said while shaking her head in disbelief.

"This is how the Temple Journey feels," I said. "It activates our sixth sense and we communicate and know things in ways we don't in this reality. The journey reminds us who we really are and how we operate when our physical senses are shut down." I smiled at her.

"So now I wait for my necklace to show up in this reality?" Denise asked.

"Yes. You'll journey to the Temple World for a few minutes a day, then go about your day-to-day life, being open to finding the necklace unexpectedly."

"What if I don't find it?" Denise asked.

"I want you to think about 'What if I do?' instead."

"So, I shouldn't worry about *not* finding it?" Denise asked.

"That's right. I'm going to ask you to just trust the journey and let it unfold as it will. We only need a small part of you to believe that you can find it. And pay attention to that belief more than any others."

"Okay, I will. I'm so excited to go see what happens. Thank you so much for this experience, Christina."

"I'm so excited for *you*, Denise," I said.

What Will You Experience?

In this chapter you will experience two significant parts of the Temple Journey. One is the meeting with your Super Watcher, which is about shedding the body you occupy in your everyday life within the 3-D world and unveiling the presence, the being behind your eyes. You're used to connecting to your physical appearance—hair texture, eye color, body type—which can keep you from experiencing your inner presence. The second part of the journey is finding an object inside the Temple, which you will later discover back in your everyday life as well. Both meeting your Super Watcher and finding your Temple World object in this reality will help to further separate you from this 3-D world so you can access and see the invisible even better.

I choose to introduce you to your Super Watcher in this chapter because when you enter the Temple World and are asked to move yourself out of your body, your brain is better able to perceive you as weightless, moving without the barrier of gravity. It has the capacity to perceive you as your higher self, the part of you that has all the answers because it doesn't reside inside a world with the rules and regulations, obstacles and barriers of our 3-D world. Then this weightless part of you eagerly seeks to find the proof that all that is inside the Temple is also a part of the third dimension, your seemingly physical reality. You will experience a lot of excitement with this journey. You will also step further away from your ego.

In the Temple World, you're not bound by the ego or

the identity you're used to having. The Super Watcher is all-knowing and lives outside time and space without limit. It occupies both your body and the invisible world of the Temple. In other words, it's the part of you that's everywhere—inside and outside of the Temple World. It knows everything about your existence and is a part of the universe, or cosmos—whatever you want to call it.

On the Super Watcher Journey, you'll connect to the timeless part of you, and that part will connect with your beloved. After this journey, you'll discover that the Temple World is not only a place you visit but a place that is a continuation of your everyday life. How? By finding the same object you discovered in the Temple World in the 3-D world. Your brain will start to back off from rejecting the Temple World. The two worlds are connected, even though it doesn't seem that they coexist. But before we go there, let's take a step back and look at this from a place of simple discovery of what it means to be alive and dead at the same time, and how science and divinity are truly connected.

The Discovery

As you know by now, after my husband died, I sought to find the truth about death. Instead, I found the meaning of life. In my pursuit of finding what comes after death, I discovered the dying inside our living. It was simple: death leads us back to life; life leads us to death. I discovered something I didn't expect, in someplace I never expected: I found divinity in science. The deeper I looked, inside the atoms, protons, molecules, and all theories and experiments and possibilities, there it was: miracles. Every day unexpected moments full of wonder. We call them miracles because we think they're not normal or frequent experiences. But there's nothing rare about these miracles. They happen all the time.

Imagine this: life is both physical and nonphysical. Those who die, die only for a moment in this reality. In the reality of their consciousness, which persists beyond time, they move to another reality, another world. The other realities, other worlds, are connected to ours. There's a presence inside us—our Super Watcher—that makes us aware of these other worlds. This presence exists in all realities, all dimensions, along with all the people you've loved and lost. To experience these other realities, you just have to learn to see with your eyes closed.

In this book, I'm asking you to consider the possibility of a reality without a physical construction. Without what we've created as a time constraint. One you must navigate without using your senses. To do so, you must access a nonphysical form from within you, your Super Watcher, to go beyond your senses and cross over as you did last week and, now, go beyond that threshold. I'm asking you to believe, truly, that you can exit this physical reality when you close your eyes and choose to go where you have not intentionally gone before.

Our "real" life isn't as we perceive it to be. It's inside a world without gravity and without the depth that we perceive. It's inside a flat surface. But we see it as a 3-D experience. How is this even possible? And why does it matter? The answer to the first question lies in the holographic universe theory.[1] Recently, scientists have found increasing evidence that the entire universe is encoded on a flat surface and that our perceived 3-D reality is a projection from the 2-D reality. In other words, our physical reality is an illusion. Our brain constructs our reality by interpreting frequencies from a reality that is in another dimension outside time and space. Our brain is an interpreter, and it's interpreting a universe that is holographic. The best way I can illustrate this concept is with the example of 3-D glasses in a movie theater. The glasses take the image from the flat screen and make it three-dimensional. We live inside the flat screen, but it feels as though we live outside it. We're here to experience this 3-D reality, which is a projection from a 2-D experience—just like in the movies when we're wearing the 3-D glasses!

To answer my second question—"Why does it matter?"—once you truly embrace that we live in a holographic universe, your Temple Journeys will become even more meaningful. They will feel—and are—as real as this everyday reality you're living in. When you can look up from this book and accept that what you see in front of you is more of an illusion than a concrete reality, then the journey you experience inside the Temple World gets to become either equally significant or at least more real than you thought it might be.

Ultimately, when you narrow everything down, we live all the way inside the molecules, the atoms, and the photons. There's so much there. Inside this flat surface where all this lives—it's all a vibration and a projection. Our consciousness and brain project this reality.

How does this relate to the Temple World? Let's look at Denise's Super Watcher Journey, where she saw the necklace with three blue stones. By sharing the description of the necklace with our class, she projected it into 3-D reality. Here's how it works. On her journey, she observed the necklace, which placed it inside her consciousness. She then transferred that experience onto the 2-D surface, and the brain brought it, as we see below, into 3-D.

Denise brought her object into her everyday life. Two weeks after she first saw the necklace, she was traveling for work. As she left her hotel room where she'd been staying the past few days, she spotted a necklace behind the Door, underneath a tiny stool. It was very similar to the one in her Temple.

"At first I felt a little confused by this," she told the class, "but then just a second later I felt joy, the kind of joy I feel inside the Temple World. I handed in the necklace at the front desk to be returned to the person who'd lost it. It wasn't my necklace to keep but my proof to remember that it is all connected. But I wonder what the necklace meant and why I saw it inside the Temple. Was Dave trying to tell me something? I can't wait to go back and ask. I can't wait to see Dave again." A lot of the times you'll have questions similar to Denise's, and often you'll find answers. And sometimes you won't, or not immediately. As you'll see in this chapter, it's possible to bring back into this experience here our beloveds, too. After all, there is no "there"; it's all here, right by your side. Your beloveds, yourself, the Temple World, even the whole universe. I bet I have your attention now, don't I?

Denise's journey illustrates that the experience of the Temple Journey impacts our lives here. If the Temple resides where thought lives, where energy lives, where information lives, and where all particles live, then just like thoughts translate into matter, the Temple World experience, which takes place at a higher vibrational place of thought, gets translated to this reality as well. You also come back with the joy you experience inside the Temple World, and it stays with you for a while here in the 3-D world. It does fade, but it lasts longer and longer the more we experience the Temple World. And when you find an object inside the Temple World, then find it here in the 3-D reality—that on its own will change the way you see the world. Finally, your interaction with your beloved, your new relationship with him or her, will change the way you feel and live here.

The good news is that what takes place inside the Temple World is free of beliefs and negative talk and is full of joy and peace—all of which translate into a beautiful 3-D experience as it passes from the 2-D surface. In other words, we can't feel negative thoughts and feelings in the Temple World, which is a shortcut. A hack. A way in to our higher self, or Super Watcher, outside false negative talk and old feelings of feeling stuck.

The Temple World takes us inside infinity, where all information lives as well as our beloved. The 3-D experience is an illusion. Death, therefore, is an illusion. You and I are even an illusion. What you have always thought to be imagination or dreams might be where we really come from. Or where the projection of us comes from. For now, let me show you how you vibrate, as that is what we are—vibrations inside a flat surface. And that is what your beloved was, and still is now.

You Are String

The holographic universe is a principle of string theory. What is string theory? Theoretical physicist, mathematician, and string theorist Brian Greene describes the basic premise in this way: "The fundamental particles of the universe that physicists have identified—electrons, neutrinos, quarks, and so on—are the 'letters' of all matter. Just like their linguistic counterparts, they appear to have no further internal substructure. String theory proclaims otherwise. According to string theory, if we could examine these particles with even greater precision—a precision many orders of magnitude beyond our present technological capacity—we would find that each is not point like, but instead consists of a tiny one-dimensional loop. Like an infinitely thin rubber band, each particle contains a vibrating, oscillating, dancing filament that physicists have named a string."[2] According to string theory, if we could see pure energy, it would look like vibrating strings of light. These dancing strings connect everything we experience. They are also what the cosmos is composed of, including ourselves. They connect us to the cosmos.

If we could see these strings, there's a very good chance we'd see one flowing from each of us all the way deep into space—a superhighway connecting us to our divine presence or higher self: our Super Watcher. You, too, will find your Super Watcher on the other end of this string.

That consciousness on the other end of that vibrating string of light and energy is the timeless part of you. Even if it's coming across as a guide or an angel or even our soul, it's all one and the same. It's all coming from Source. We can interact with this consciousness. This interaction bypasses the 3-D hologram. It bypasses death. I know these are bold statements, but there is no halfway to this truth. We either believe that we live beyond this concrete reality or we don't. The Temple World is created as the gateway to knowing an existence without death, the missing piece to the larger reality.

The Super Watcher is more like metaconsciousness that's between lives and between worlds. It's a vital part of our evolution and growth. It's the part that connects us to our life outside of the projection. In the Temple Journey, you get to interact with those you've lost, and bringing in a "separate self"—in the form of the Super Watcher—helps us experience these higher dimensions in what I call the Temple World. Our understanding of that separate self is vital in this journey. This seemingly separate self is the truest part of you that begins to fade experientially when your 3-D experience begins at birth. You want to slowly bring back this core part and name it Super Watcher so your brain can start to observe it and bring it into your projection. In other words, or in words that better fit this reality, the Super Watcher is the guide you'll get to talk with, share your insights with, and feel guided by.

But the farther we go on this journey, the louder the Survivor voice will get. When we're able to quiet the Survivor, which is part of the 3-D engine, we become much more able to exit this reality. We can let go of our limiting beliefs and start fully connecting with our Super Watcher. On this journey, your first after the Door, you will meet your Super Watcher.

The human self, our persona in this reality, finds it hard to believe that it has access to such extraordinary information, and therefore that self has an easier time receiving information if it believes it comes from a higher source outside the self. Simply put, our guides, angels, and saints are all part of us, and we all have access to them, to ourselves. The brain loves the naming, the labeling, and the dividing from self, but ultimately we all are one.

There Is No Separation

Even people who are open to the possibility of life beyond this life speak about it, they tend to use a very simplistic way to describe how our loved ones who have died connect with us: "He's watching over you" or "She's always with you." Though these statements are true, they place you *outside* the experience, a passive recipient of this attention. The implication is that you may not even feel or sense that your loved one is watching you. You're not being told that you can actively connect to your loved one, to a higher power, a source of light and divinity.

That's why grief is so painful. Because we feel we're separated from our loved one who's died in this reality, the loved ones we feel are a huge part of who we are. The self that lives inside the vibration, inside consciousness. The projection to 3-D makes us look and feel separate, and this causes deep pain. We yearn to be with them. We yearn to see them. Why? Because we have always belonged together. And this projection makes it seem as if we never will be again. Not true.

There is so much more to the way our beloveds are with us than those old sayings meant to comfort allow. Our loved ones are connected with us in ways that don't seem to be real from the 3-D perspective. Well-intended words such as "They're always with you" and "They're watching over you" are true, but they don't bring depth and understanding to the bereaved; they're simplified versions of a much vaster world that coexists alongside us. Understanding that world, finding our way there, and navigating through it bring meaning and understanding to these old phrases.

But too often, when we try to step outside the preconceived and limited perception of what happens after we die, of who we really are (eternal beings, eternal consciousness), we come up against judgment and shame, not only from the people around us, but also from inside ourselves. We're preconditioned to believe that death is real and that nothing exists beyond what we can perceive with our five senses. But now I tell you that you're a vibrating string of light connecting to another vibrating string of light, which is your higher divine self. I mean, yes, this sounds really out there. But it really isn't. Think about waves of light. Or sound. We accept these as facts. It's not so different. My hope is the fact that how we perceive our experience is an illusion will allow you to open yourself to a new possibility of truth.

As you can see, we're starting to experience new ideas, feelings, sensations, and realities through this book, but we always come back to live in this physical reality. This is where we need to be. No matter how far away we travel and how blissful and beautiful the worlds we visit, we actually experience our lives right here, on planet Earth. Ultimately, we come back here. We always return to this projection of reality, and that's okay. Nothing wrong with that. We're meant to experience life from here for now. But that doesn't mean we shouldn't know that it's a projection, a filtering experience from the brain, and a labeling experience from the human egoic self.

You Exist Inside *and* Outside Your Body

When you meet your Super Watcher for the first time, your brain—the origin of that human egoic self—might try to put your consciousness inside your body because that's where it thinks it lives. You, your consciousness, *is* inside this body, but you also exist outside your body. The same goes for the people we've lost. To connect with what we cannot see and hear, and with those who've left their bodies, we must let go of the idea of being contained inside our bodies. This is no easy task. The life of the body is deeply convincing—we're in this body to experience the physical reality and learn from these experiences.

But before you were inside this body, you were inside the universe and connected to the all, in unity consciousness. This connection does not go away; it just gets quieter over time. The vibrating light string continues to hold you next to and part of everyone else, including the person you lost from this physical reality, which is why, for the rest of this book, for the most part, I'll be avoiding the use of "dead" or "death" when referring to your loved one who is no longer with us in this physical reality.

Once one particle in the universe is connected to another, they can never be disconnected. Even if they're miles and miles apart, galaxies apart. This connection of particles is called quantum entanglement. In his book *The Holographic Universe*, Michael Talbot, one of the greatest metaphysics writers of our time, explains that near-death experiences, or death, is really nothing more—listen to this—than the shifting of the person's consciousness from one level of the hologram of reality to another.[3] The fact that the people we think we lost are just in a different reality in the hologram, and that we can connect with them if we want to, are beyond anything I could have imagined on my own when my husband left this physical reality. I wish someone had told me this. And showed me how to connect.

We must also let go of the idea that source is not part of us. We are not only the projected. We are the projector. We are not only the created but the creators. We are not only the seer but also the seen. Many biologists believe that human consciousness, self-awareness, emerged to speed up the brain's problem-solving mechanism. These scientists believe that material existence and its demands evolved consciousness.[4] In other words, consciousness came after existence. In this book, the premise is that consciousness came first, followed by the rest of the universe, because it was created by our observations—how we interpreted what we experienced. We were the ones projecting our consciousness and creating matter. Nothing in this world exists without an observer. Nothing is created without a witness to the creation. You are the observer, the witness. You get to determine which universe to create in 3-D.

The steps you'll take on this journey are going to be enough to give you not only knowledge about our universe but also a way to access that universe, which in truth belongs to you. You created it. You made it happen. Yes, you. I know this sounds a little too much, but it's true. You are the creator of galaxies and suns. You are the observer of many moons and black holes. You and your Super Watcher that's connected to Source, that *is* Source, observed life, and created life. All you're doing on this Temple Journey is remembering that you're the creator and that you have access to those realms, to all parts of the hologram.

Our version of reality is created by our belief in it. Our observation of it allows for one of the many worlds that are possible to come through to the 3-D world. We will talk about the many worlds interpretation theory a little farther down in our journey. But for now, what you need to understand is that when I discuss setting an intention, I mean focusing on one specific desired outcome. This will collapse all other possible outcomes and it will influence the course of our reality. When we find a specific object inside our Temple Journey, and we carry its image and our experience of it back into this reality, we indirectly tell our consciousness to look for it in our 3-D experiences.

For example, when Denise observed the necklace with the blue stones, it entered her brain and collapsed the other possibilities— different necklace, no necklace, and infinite versions of both. Through her observation, she projected the necklace into the 3-D reality. When she returned from the journey, her brain sought to find the necklace in the physical reality even when she wasn't consciously looking. The Temple Journeys give the brain new visuals, new neural network connections, and when we're in this physical reality, these connections create a need to find the object, because the brain thinks it's real. And why do we need to find an object, or create anything from inside the Temple World? Because if it's true that the Temple World is as real as the 3-D world, and connected with the 3-D world, then you'll have the proof you need to believe that your beloved you encountered inside the Temple World is real, too. And as with the object, in many ways we get to bring them back with us. After all, they never really left. They only stopped appearing in the third dimension with their physical bodies. But they're still inside the holographic universe, hanging out in a different part of it, waiting for us to find them. I dare you. I dare you to believe in this truth and find your way to your beloved.

Human thought does determine reality. Now that we know this, now that we're beginning to believe it, imagine what we could do. We could live without fear, or with much less of it. We could be timeless, despite the age of our body, realizing it's only our temporary home and our consciousness isn't confined to it. We could overcome grief in a less self-destructive way. We could evolve our human species in ways we experience only in the most uplifting science fiction books and movies. Maybe we could even begin to experience a life without death in it. I know what I'm proposing is bold and daring, but grief isn't for the faint of heart, and you're working through it. And if you're not dealing with loss, and you're just excited about what happens after we die and living a more expansive reality, you had the courage and spirit to pick up this book. So if anyone can dare to push their reality beyond its past limitations, it's you.

I say "beginning" to believe because it will take a lot of proof for the brain to accept as fact that human thought determines reality. Even if you feel that you believe it now, while reading this book or in your Temple Circle, once you go back into your everyday life and everyday world, you'll be deeply influenced by this 3-D reality. We get pulled back in. We even forget about the proof we found along the way. The brain dismisses proof unless it's repeated many times. Often, people see the miraculous or seemingly illogical for themselves, but because nobody else has seen what they have, or they've seen something miraculous only once, they'll dismiss their own experience. I bet you've dismissed miraculous and illogical things such as synchronistic moments. That's what we do, until we don't.

Maybe Christopher Columbus sailing across the ocean felt the same way you feel about believing there's something out there beyond what you can see. He *had* to get to the other side of the world, as he understood it, because he believed. There are times in history that we've taken big leaps of faith, and they paid off. Connecting with the divine part of you, the Super Watcher, is one of those times. All you'll be doing on the Temple Journey is remembering that greater you. You're taking a small step toward the next frontier of your evolution. The Super Watcher will feel strange at first because you haven't been in contact with that part of you for so long, especially if you've gone through loss, but once you feel connected to this part, it will feel like coming home. It's your home, after all.

One of the emotions you'll experience as you activate your Super Watcher on this journey is increasing certainty, until one day you'll forget your doubtfulness about the nonphysical world and remember your wisdom. You'll reconnect with who you've always been and always will be—a source of knowing and love. I know these words sound so basic, but ultimately the messages I've received from my journeys to the Temple World have been about love, happiness, and just pure joy. That is what we are underneath all the doubt and the worry and, of course, underneath all the pain—we are beings of love, light, and joy. Your Super Watcher will guide you in remembering this.

The Super Watcher evolved from the Watcher, whom I introduced in my book *Second Firsts*. The Watcher self is a voice of reason, logic, and timeless wisdom. The Super Watcher is not a part of the 3-D world, or even confined inside your brain. It is an intergalactic, interstellar traveler who has been a part of your many life experiences. If the Watcher is wisdom, the Super Watcher is God, source, divinity. If the Watcher is knowing what to do with your life, the Super Watcher is being the stillness, the energy inside the Field.

Now, whenever I doubt myself, I walk inside my Temple World, connect with my Super Watcher, and I'm immediately reminded of my own divinity. The Temple World is a church that was built in the universe, and the Super Watcher is the divinity that created this place so you could experience joy. And since the Super Watcher is your highest self that comes from Source, it's you who created the Temple World and it's you who chose to experience life in it. You're reading these pages because you've asked for this book and this journey. You're reading because you've found your way to your own voice.

Meeting Your Beloved

You might be wondering when you're supposed to meet your beloved for the first time on this Temple Journey. As you saw from the previous chapter, many people meet with them immediately, which, as I've said, surprised me. This rapid connection speaks to the readiness of our brain to allow for that to happen. It also speaks to how ready our beloveds are to be visited. But you've only begun. If you met your beloved as soon as you walked through the Door, meeting your Super Watcher—and finding your object—is still critical to make this experience a long-term part of your life. It's a deeper journey, more difficult to doubt—when the 3-D world wants to take the higher dimensions away from you and keep you inside the illusion of its existence.

I'm referring to our brain and its automatic nature to bring us "back to reality" against all odds. The deeper we go inside the Temple World, the stronger and easier the connection with your beloved will be. Imagine living your life in 3-D in the future and spending a few minutes a day connected to the invisible world that is part of you and making that a natural part of your day. This is how I live my life now. I close my eyes a few minutes a day and transport myself there. So stay with me and the teachings of this book even if you've already connected with your beloved and found your proof. We're just getting started.

Some of the very first people who traveled inside the Temple World were my children. My fifteen-year-old daughter, Isabel, shared with me in writing what took place in one of her Temple World visits, where she saw her dad for the first time. Reading her experience was incredibly emotional for me. Isabel was only four years old when her father passed away and, a few years into her grieving journey, she requested to see a therapist, articulating a desire to talk with—as she said—a "stranger" about her loss. Losing her dad was and still is the most impactful and difficult experience of her life.

She saw the school's counselor and got a lot out of this experience, but she always sought to find him. She always asked me if Daddy was watching over her. She was also the one who drew his ghost often and made the ghost part of her family drawings after his passing. As the years went by, this part of her was no longer present. She stopped talking about ghosts and no longer drew them. When Isabel took the Super Watcher Journey, she was fifteen years old, ten years after she drew the ghost pictures.

She was extremely eager to go inside the Temple World. We picked a day to take the journey together, and when that day came, she said with an almost impatient voice, "Mommy, I'm ready. Let's go." We lay down on the bed, closed our eyes, held hands, put on the Temple sound, and I guided her just as I'm guiding all of you.

Isabel wanted me to add her experience to this book so you could read it, too. Here's Isabel's journey in her exact words.

My Super Watcher drops me off at this little island where if I look right and left, I can see the ocean at all equal distances.

The island was a perfect oval.

When I look in front of me, I see trees, not tropical, just regular trees that are five feet above my head.

I walk down two steps that lead me to the ground that had no trees or grass. The area forms a perfect circle about three meters in diameter and is made of a tan smooth rock.

I realize that this is the exact "island" that was shown on Avatar: The Last Airbender, *of course, that's what my mind shows me.*

On the rock-like surface, there are markings that create many circles following the perimeter, like a mandala, but not as detailed. They were very faint gray markings with small triangles that outline the circles following the perimeter.

In the middle of the paved circle, I see a red box.

I open the red box to see a small red jewelry bag, only instead of jewelry, it contains gray pebbles with darker gray spots on them.

Once I look up from the bag, I see a figure making his way through the trees straight ahead of me, and he makes his way onto the circle.

I look straight up, and just like my Super Watcher, he is all white. I quickly realize it is my father who makes his way out of the trees and stands two meters away from me.

He smiles as I go to hug him.

It made me happy, but I was not crying or jumping around in excitement. I just hugged him and felt happy. I think the reason I wasn't sobbing or crying was because I had imagined this moment in my head all the time.

I see Daddy by my side and I know he is with me at all times, either walking with me during school or looking after me from above. It felt normal and I was glad that I could see him. He is still white for some reason, just like my Super Watcher. He kneels down and I see I have grown smaller, turning into my four-year-old self.

He tells me how he is so proud of me about track and tae kwon do and how I am so smart. I remember this is how he used to talk to me. He would be on one knee and at face level, speaking. I tell him I miss him and he says he knows and that he misses us, too.

When I write that Daddy and I are having a conversation, we weren't really talking or moving our mouths. We just kind of knew, speaking with our minds like we have been for the past eleven years. Through this conversation I get a memory that I don't realize I was getting until after I "woke up" from the Temple. My mother has told me that when I was a baby, he would hold me in the bed and we would fall asleep. He in a way delivered this memory to me and I didn't realize that he was until fully analyzing my experience with him afterward.

We say good bye and I leave with my Super Watcher. I have had many other experiences with my father in the Temple World since then—when I've been stressed or something happens and I am having a hard time, we would play in the stars together and feel the energy the universe was providing us. It was a peaceful and enjoyable feeling seeing my father again. Not overwhelming or "too much to handle." I was happy I could fully see him and experience that world with him.

I can't tell you how thrilled I was for my daughter to have this experience. It brought her such excitement, happiness, and peace. It became a safe place for her to visit. Her relationship with her dad is much different than it would have been without her taking the journey. And because of that she is more at peace about her dad's passing. Even though she still questions it all, she's able to be more at peace in her everyday life as a teen.

When I talk about having a relationship with the person who has died it may come across as silly or impossible. But because of what I learned from this journey and the science that tells us about the holographic universe, the many world interpretations, and the many other dimensions we can't see with the naked eye, I believe that our beloveds are still alive—just without their bodies. We can have a relationship with them and talk to them without being perceived as if we've lost our minds. What we've lost is the limited view of our reality.

I'm asking a lot from you in this book. I understand that. In a way, I'm asking you to break through the walls of this illusion and find your way into another dimension, one without time. One without your body being with you, and one where nobody is ever dead. Now it's your turn to meet your divinity, your Super Watcher, and find your way to a life-changing experience, just as Isabel did.

The Super Watcher Journey

When I first went inside the Temple World to meet my Super Watcher and observe what that presence looked like, I was sure

I was going to see a human form, because my brain said I would see another version of me. But that's not how it appeared to me. There was only light. An orb. In later journeys, the orb changed to an eagle, and now it's a constellation of stars in the dark sky that comes down to speak to me and be with me. The more I visited my Super Watcher, the more I evolved, and the more I evolved, the more it evolved into its pure form.

Now this constellation serves as my guides. They come and greet me as soon as I go through the Door and take me with them inside the Temple World. I feel surrounded by light and source. Your Super Watcher could look like a glowing light, a person, a flower, a bird, a star, a feather. Really anything. Pay attention to what you see and trust it.

The first time you meet your Super Watcher is always so special. How often do you get to meet your consciousness? How often do you consciously bring in a guide to walk alongside you, a guide that's yours, timeless? This guide has been with you all along, and when you meet them the first time, know that you have met many times before. Trust your experience. Trust the journey; don't let the Survivor take that away from you. Remember, you're in a safe environment where you're always in control.

If for some reason you *don't* see your Super Watcher the first time you try, that's okay. You can go back whenever you're ready, as many times as you want or need. There's no right or wrong. Everyone's journey is unique, just as your thoughts and the way you look at the world are completely individual. I also can't wait for you to find your first object, one of my very favorite moments.

THROUGH THE PORTAL

Find a comfortable chair in a quiet place where you won't be disturbed. Read the instructions once or twice before you close your eyes to take the journey. Remember to have something on hand—a notebook, an iPad, etc.—to record your experience after the journey. If you'd like, you can play the corresponding sound vibration or other music, or simply proceed in silence. Relax your shoulders. You're in a safe space.

1. Take a deep breath and release. Take another deep breath and with that second breath look within you, beyond the darkness of your closed eyes.

2. Travel through the darkness and toward your Door.

3. The Door might be identical to the first time you went through or it might be a different Door altogether. Look at its colors, experience the feelings you get as you approach the Door. When you reach the Door, cross the threshold.

4. Feel the shift in the air around you, the increase in vibrations, the leaving behind of this 3-D reality. Feel yourself entering another dimension where this journey exists, which you feel in your heart as deep joy and peace. As you feel this dimension, tell your brain that you're accessing a deeper place where you're vibrating at a higher frequency, where your existence is made up of patterns and a vibrating string of light.

5. Now look around and get ready to meet your Super Watcher. You're going to feel its presence inside your body first. Slowly and very gently move your consciousness out of your body. See your consciousness transferring from you until it's right next to you, connected by a vibrating string of light. This is a safe experience for your brain. As you guide your consciousness out of your body this first time, it slowly takes shape. Observe what it looks like. How big or small is it? How does it communicate with you? If it's a light or ball of light, what color is it? If it's a tree, what kind? However it manifests, pay attention and observe it closely. Your consciousness is different from everyone else's and you'll have a different visual experience from anyone else. This is your Super Watcher.

6. Walk farther away from the Door with your Super Watcher by your side.

7. When you look directly in front of you now you see a spinning Portal. An entryway into another world. It's beautiful and it's safe. Know that it could be a square opening. It could be a circle. It could be anything you want it to be. This Portal is going to take you beyond time and space.

8. Enter the Portal with your Super Watcher. You're transported into a beautiful, mesmerizing galaxy of stars. You are now moving faster than the speed of light. Look around you and see the stars and all the galaxies you're passing by.

9. You have arrived at the other side of the Portal, and step out into a new place. This place could be anywhere—on another planet, on a star, on the moon, in Hawaii, or in the Milky Way.

10. Look around and familiarize yourself with your environment. What do you see? With your Super Watcher by your side, scan the area and notice who is there. Is your beloved there, waving at you? Are there other people there? Strangers or familiar faces? Take it all in. You're deep inside the most incredible place, a journey unlike any other journey you've taken. A place where everyone you have lost exists. If you see your beloved, allow for that experience to take place. Go to him or her. Take time being with your loved one.

11. Bask in this experience. Stay here for as long as you want. Take in all the feelings you are feeling. Your emotions. Your tears. Your laughter. This is an extraordinary moment.

THE OBJECT

1. Now, as you're standing or sitting with your beloved and your Super Watcher, look around for a small object. It will be something you can pick up and bring back with you. Stay in this peaceful experience and be open to finding whatever the object might be. However unexpected it may be. Get close to what you find and touch it. Pick it up and hold it in your hands. Look at it from every angle. Know that you get to bring this back with you. What have you found? Feel the substance of it. Is it soft? Is it tough? Is it smooth or shiny? Does

it have a crack, a spot of color? And how does it make you feel to hold it, to see it?

2. Start walking back toward the Portal while holding fast to your object. Your Super Watcher is right here walking with you. Look around one more time. Remember this place. Say good-bye to your beloved. You'll see each other again soon. Say good-bye to anyone else who has met you here, and make your way back. You're going to reenter the Portal you came through. And we're going to go all the way back to the Door. Look at the galaxies, the stars, the sky. It's so beautiful. Take notice of your Super Watcher right next to you.

3. The Portal has brought you back to where you first met your Super Watcher. Look at your Super Watcher and smile and ask for your consciousness to come back to you the way your brain understands this concept, to feel that it's inside your body. Slowly feel your consciousness and your presence come back into your body. It's always part of you and it's also always somewhere everywhere—else.

4. Holding the object in your hand, walk toward the Door, go through it and back to your place here in this reality. Now slowly take a deep breath and gently bring yourself back to this reality. Welcome back from your second journey.

5. This is the time to write down everything you saw and experienced. Your first moment with your Super Watcher, going

through the Portal, your time with your beloved on the other side of the Portal and what you got to bring back.

Where Did You Go?

Every journey takes us deeper and deeper into the universe. Closer to Source and to our true timeless being. With each journey, we'll get closer to our Super Watcher and the people we love and lost. You'll get to experience moments that you'll question when you come back. That's part of the journey. Remember that your Survivor never likes to take time off, especially when you're going so far outside your comfort zone. These passages you went through—the Door, the Portal—are real. They exist in the universe. You went through and found yourself in a brand-new location.

You also found something special. You held on to it. And you brought it back with you. The reason I asked you to bring something back with you is fundamental to this journey—this is your object. From my experience, your Super Watcher will look for your object in your everyday reality and show it to you. The only way for you to create a new reality is to convince your brain that this is possible and that it's true. When I first started, when I had my doubts, I would test myself by doing this exercise. It involves taking a big risk because you could come back and say you didn't find your object anywhere. What would that mean? But I was willing to take that risk. I hope you are, too.

One of my students, Laura, could not find her object at first, though she kept searching. "My first object was a round, white 'ball.' I couldn't find it for days and I would pick up anything that was round to see if it matched (as in random things I found on the road). I found a picture that was very close, really spot on, but I wanted something more concrete. Finally my husband said, 'Laura, that looks like the moon.' Wow . . . yes, the picture looked like the moon. I loved it and felt much better. I mean, what could be better? Since then I have discovered the gemstone moonstone and I'm going to have a necklace made so I can wear one all the time."

My student Carrie also found that her object appeared in a way she didn't expect, but which affected her profoundly: "My object was an old-fashioned key and it took me some time to find it. Interestingly, my time in the Temple World has been focused on my work—because I worked so closely with my husband, I wasn't sure what I wanted to do when he passed. I have had to make many decisions about my work, the building we owned together, and dealing with offers of other possibilities since his death. One day at my office while talking with my assistant I was leaning against a wall that gave me a different perspective of the office. I saw a painting a friend had given us when we bought the office, and in the painting is the key—it's physically embedded in the painting. It made me so happy and gave me the sense that I am going in the right direction." While Carrie recounted her experience, I think I felt as blown away as she was. Each time we connect our day-to-day reality with the Temple World it's an incredible experience.

"My object was a rock," said Sandy. "I remember that I happened to find it in a glass box on my dresser. The box has been there forever and it contained shells and dried flowers from past adventures but also rocks from Lake Superior. The box was right there, front and center. I'd never noticed it before. Most of the rocks were on the bottom. I was moving a jewelry box that was blocking the box of shells and it just caught my eye. I placed it in a little pouch and now carry it with me for good luck and just to hold when I need that connection."

Another favorite story of mine is Cherrie's: "My first object was a purple ball of yarn. I remember during the Temple Journey I saw it at my feet, laying in a grassy field, and I was like 'What's this?' I thought I would never find a ball of purple yarn, as yarn is just not in my scope of daily interests, I mean I'm not a yarn girl at all. I didn't find my purple ball of yarn right away. It took me a few weeks, actually. I found a brown ball of yarn one day while I was volunteering at the Humane Society—a cat toy, but not purple, and I remember posting to the group about that, and you said to me 'You are getting closer.' I think that validation of 'getting closer' helped *a lot*. Another week went by and I was visiting my daughter at college, in another town, with no idea of what activities we might do. We were walking along the sidewalk about to go into a coffee shop and right there, next to the entrance of the café, is a yarn shop, with a display of balls of yarn in the window and there is my purple ball of yarn. I grabbed my daughter's arm and pulled her in. The dots connected for me that day."

When you find your object in this reality after discovering it in the Temple World, your brain will start to create a new belief, a belief that what you get to experience in the other reality—all the goodness, the insights, and the new life—you can have here, too. Similarly, every time you have a conversation with your beloved, bring those moments back with you. There is no veil. No wall. No gap between here and there.

And if you believe that, you believe that you're the creator of your world. When your mind opens that gateway into a world of creation, life and grief will never be the same. Of course, opening yourself to that world takes practice, perseverance. The holographic theory says that the projection is what's created in the two-dimensional world. That's where we need to be to create. We don't create here. Here is hard work. We read slowly. We write slowly. We cook slowly. We clean the floor slowly. We grieve slowly. And there is nothing wrong with that. But we also reenter slowly. We lose life because of grief. And our souls are here to experience living and creating.

Your Homework for This Week

First and foremost, take the journey from the beginning to this point every day. Even if you have only a few minutes to spend. Go through the Door, meet your Super Watcher, experience the divine voice, experience the presence of your Super Watcher, and with that presence, look for your beloved. Every day. Then, with your beloved and your Super Watcher, take the journey through the Portal into the stars and through the galaxy. When you're on the other side, continue any conversations with your beloved, feel the essence of your consciousness, your Super Watcher, as much as possible and spend time with your object. Then bring it back.

This week is about finding your object in your reality here. And experiencing the surprise and joy when suddenly, out of the blue, the object shows up at work, in a store, among a pile of things in your closet that you haven't looked through in ages. When you find it, take a picture of it, and write down what it felt like when your object showed up. Also tell someone in your Temple Circle, or if you don't have anyone you've told about this journey, this may be a good time to tell one person. Talking about your experience makes it stronger in this reality.

Having something show up here that you saw in the Temple World is a big deal, so you want to record and cement that experience so the pathways your brain creates for this occurrence are as strong as possible. We're building an entire network of pathways throughout this journey, and each occurrence of a miracle in our journeys deepens the automatic ability of the brain to allow miracles to happen daily, spontaneously. This will open the Doors to exciting, synchronistic experiences, moments where you're reminded of the Temple World as a regular occurrence. It will open the Door to more objects and experiences that are part of the Temple Journey to find their way to the life you are living now.

Laura, who found her object to be the moon and wanted it transformed into a moonstone necklace to carry with her every day, shared with me that she began experiencing many moments of synchronicity. For example, she would be reading a book and certain words would jump out that connected her to her Temple Journey. She's still not quite used to it, and she sometimes wonders if her brain's seeking these moments deliberately. She made sure to tell me that she's determined to find a white moon-like crystal ball randomly in a store, at a friend's, wherever she will stumble upon it, she is certain of it. She deeply believes that it will happen eventually—as it always does. And that knowing is the programming and rewiring that the Temple World experiences allow for.

Congratulations on daring to go deeper into this journey of invisible worlds that only come to life when we trust ourselves to experience what is not seen by the naked eye. You made contact with your beloved by your visiting with them instead of them coming to visit with you. You guided your brain to let go of your physical body and find your way to the consciousness and being of the person you lost from your 3-D world. This is a big deal. And you must be so proud of yourself for overriding the illusion of this dimension and finding your way to another side of the holographic universe to a place where death and dying are never real. You let this version of yourself go so a new way of looking at the world could come forth. Human evolution happens only when we want to understand our reality and go beyond what lies in front of us. And you did just that. You also saw yourself as you really are. Timeless. Ageless. Outside time and space. A part of a universe of vibrating strings of light. Where, in a sense, you're not alive either. When you seek to go inside the Temple World, you and your beloved are in the same experience. Beyond the third dimension.

the temple of universes

Now let me sit here, on the threshold of two worlds.

Lost in the eloquence of silence.

—JALALUDDIN RUMI

I cried when I saw my Miraculous Universe for the first time," Julia said as she burst into nervous laughter. She kept shaking her head as if to dismiss what she saw.

"Tell us all about it," I said to her—and before I even finished my words she started sharing about the sea breeze that came through the bedroom window at her beach house. "I knew I was with someone special in that house, but I don't know who. I also knew that my kids were at the beach in front of the house. I don't know how I knew, but I did. And my son was there with them, playing with my daughters." Julia had lost her first child, her son, over a decade earlier. He was stillborn. A few years later she and her husband divorced. Julia craved finding happiness again.

"My son, Stephen, was playing with my daughters as if he had always been there," Julia said and smiled while wiping away her tears. "Maybe next time I'll go down to the beach and play with them, too." She looked up at me immediately after saying it and asked a difficult question—one I had heard before: "What does it mean that my son is there with the girls in my Miraculous Universe?" She looked at me, anxiously awaiting my response to the most important question of all. "In this miraculous life we get to observe inside the Temple of Universes; do we also get to bring back with us the person we lost?"

"Julia, are you asking me if you could bring Stephen back?" I asked, wanting to not shy away from this question.

"Yes, I guess that's what I am asking," she said and smiled at me, not wanting to seem impatient or as if she were rejecting the journey in any way.

"Stephen has always been there waiting for you to see him. Waiting for you to know that he has never left. Now the only difference is that you both know it. You can observe this new beautiful life with the beach house, with your girls playing together with him and with this partner who is at your home, someone you have yet to meet," I said and paused waiting for her to take it all in.

"So I am finally seeing what has always been there, and I didn't know it. Stephen never left us, we just didn't know he was by our side," Julia said and looked away.

"That's exactly right," I said.

What Will You Experience?

If only I could show you the many versions of your life. They would appear like a million raindrops, each reflecting a different view. Dropping on you all at once. But you couldn't possibly see each of them as they hit the ground. You would have to choose which one to follow all the way to its landing. And you would choose the biggest drop, with the best, clearest reflection inside it. Wouldn't you?

This is what this chapter is about. Looking for your raindrop—bringing those you lost into your future. It is also about bringing yourself toward a future that you want. How will you do that? You will learn about the many universes and dimensions and their possible realities. Yes, there are so many. And they all belong to you. They have been yours for eternity. You just have to notice them. You just have to choose them. This is what you'll do when you visit the Temple of Universes. Imagine a place, almost like a home, where everything comes together, where all our worlds—all possible pasts, presents, futures—and all the people we love, gather. That is the Temple of Universes.

By now you are starting to embrace the possibility that death isn't real. That the person you lost is with you as you're stepping into a new chapter in your life. Knowing that can ease the pain and fear you feel and allows you to be more open to what is possible. Of course, knowing death isn't real doesn't take away the fact that you don't have the physical person you lost in *this* life—that you can't hold hands, drink coffee together, or go on a road trip with them—but it does help to know that that person still exists. And that what you experience in the Temple World is a part of our multidimensional existence.

The Multiverse Inside the Temple

What do I mean by multidimensional? Well, our universe is believed to be 95 percent invisible, or comprised of dark matter.

The remaining 5 percent or so—stars, planets, galaxies, clusters of galaxies—is observable, either to our naked eye or with the help of instruments.[1] According to our perception, that visible world, the physical world in which we live, has only three dimensions we can see—depth, height, and width. The fourth dimension, which is time, serves to move us forward, and it also holds us in that forward movement. In other words, we can't travel backward or sideways in our 3-D reality. Superstring theory suggests that there are six more dimensions, that we live inside a multiverse, in a world where many universes, as well as infinite versions of ourselves, exist.

How do these dimensions differ from the first four? Imagine a bookcase with books on it. Each book contains a whole universe. When you are in the third dimension, you are inside one of those books. You can't get out. You can't look at the bookcase from afar. You can't even imagine that there is another book next to you. You think that everything that exists is inside the book, where you are.

In the fifth dimension, you're reading the book—you can move backward and forward in time. You're not restricted to the present moment. If you are in the fifth dimension, going back in time would be as easy as walking down the street.

In the sixth dimension, you're looking at the bookcase full of books. Each book has the same beginning but different outcomes. So the initial condition of your world, your life, is the same for each universe. For example, let's say you're born in Arizona and live in a stucco house with your mom, dad, and two siblings and, because of later actions (from taking a left turn instead of a right, to majoring in engineering rather than psychology), your future timeline changes. There might be a version where you live in a different country but have the same job. A version where you have different hair and a different house. A version where you have the same house, different hair, and a new job. And the list goes on infinitely. According to theoretical astrophysics, it's completely possible.

In the seventh dimension, the initial conditions are different. For example, for each timeline, you get to be born in another country with different parents. The eighth and ninth dimensions become even more complex. The best way to understand the fifth through the ninth dimensions is to imagine that they allow for more flexibility of maneuvering yourself in different planes, with different beginnings and endings and lots of back-and-forth. You would be able to observe older and younger versions of yourself. In the tenth dimension and possibly beyond, everything is possible. Everything you can imagine.[2]

You may be wondering if it's possible to access all these dimensions when you get to the Temple of Universes. Yes. The Temple of Universes Journey will help you glimpse all the possibilities open to you. The Temple of Universes lives where all the invisible matter lies. It has intelligence. It's at the source of the universe. Where your consciousness comes from. Where your Super Watcher calls home. Where the vibrating strings originate. Where the Big Bang sparked light. Where your beloved lives every single day in infinity. Where I found my husband. Where I felt his intelligence and mind combined. Where I felt free to see beyond the limits of my physical reality and create a life that was too wild for me to imagine in this normal experience.

You're living only one version of the infinite possible universes. In the Temple of Universes everything will be at your disposal. You just have to choose what you want. That's the way it's always been. We're just used to believing in this one physical reality more than the power of our consciousness. Yet the nothingness that surrounds us is anything but. It's the arena of infinite possibilities that has been in plain sight all along.

Imagine the possibilities life holds for us if we learn to *consciously* decide to collapse the versions of reality we don't want to bring into being for ourselves and create the version we do. In the Temple of the Universes, this is exactly what will happen. You will observe multiple possible versions of your lives and choose the life you want for yourself—choose the future you want for yourself. When you choose one possibility, all the other possibilities collapse. How does this work? When we stop observing something it has less power over our 3-D reality. This is called the Observer Effect, which is one of my favorite laws.

According to Werner Heisenberg's uncertainty principle, an unobserved small object (an electron, photon, or particle of light) exists in an amorphous state, with no location, no motion. It's everywhere and nowhere. Until it's observed. As Robert Lanza explains, "Physicists describe the phantom, not-yet-manifest condition as a wave function, a mathematical expression used to find the probability that a particle will appear in any given place. When a property of an electron suddenly switches from possibility to reality, some physicists say its wave function has collapsed."[3] In the same vein, when we observe an event—a version of our lives—and choose it, the universe mirrors that choice as our reality and collapses all the other non-observed potentials.

In one of my favorite experiments, scientists assumed that light is a particle. When they observed it as such, then light was a particle. But when they did an experiment observing it as a wave, guess what happened? The light behaved as a wave. What we observe changes. What we notice is influenced by us noticing it.

Gregg Braden, a *New York Times* bestselling author who bridges science, spirituality, and human potential, says that the possibilities of our future are determined by our choices in the present.

A choice point occurs when conditions appear that create a path between the present course of events and a new course leading to new outcomes. The choice point is like a bridge making it possible to begin one path and change course to experience the outcome of a new path. . . . The tools that make such a jump possible are found in our beliefs: the thoughts, feelings, and emotions that the new reality was already in place. Choice points may occur more often than we think.[1]

It's in the spaces between thought and observation, in the silence between the pulses of creation, that we have the opportunity to "jump" from one possibility to the next. This space is where the miracles occur. In the journey you'll take in this chapter, once inside the Temple of Universes, you'll project your consciousness into the future you choose. You're attempting to slip between the present moment and the future, between the now and the moments after the now. So you can move from one choice point to the next.

Choosing Your Version of Infinite Outcomes

The Temple of Universes is the heart of the Temple Journey. You'll begin this journey as you usually do. You'll go through the Door, meet with your beloved and your Super Watcher, then travel through the Portal. As you exit the Portal, you'll see from afar a place that looks like an actual Temple, whatever that means to you. Mine is an ancient building with big pillars. Yours might be a beach house like Julia's was, a Jetsons-style home made of crystal, a floating bowling alley, or a structure you recognize from your dreams—who knows? Be open to what comes through. Each Temple is different because each person is different. Just be open to yours.

When you arrive at the Temple of Universes step inside and take your time looking around. On this first journey, your Temple will be divided into three areas, each reflecting one of your three possible outcomes. There are infinite versions of possible outcomes, and of course we can't review them all, so three is more than enough for this journey. On one side of the Temple, you'll see your status quo reality, which I call the Average Outcome Universe. On the opposite side, you'll see your fear-based reality, your Survivor outcome universe, where you worry a lot about things going wrong. Directly in front of you, between these two realities, you'll observe the miraculous version of your future. The version you can only see in your dreams.

The Average reality for me was about living alone for the rest of my life raising my children and never being in a partnership again. My average reality kept me healthy and well but without anyone by my side. My fear Survivor-based reality was that I was going to run out of money and my kids wouldn't have health insurance. I had all kinds of fears attached to that reality. I was glad to collapse it and never allow myself to observe it again. During this journey, you'll collapse the versions you don't want. You won't think any more about them. You'll focus on a possibility that feels so good it's almost a miracle. You'll look at all the details of this life so they become real in your thoughts and mind. And soon, when you're back in the 3-D world, you'll start to see this new life being created there.

After you collapse the two you don't want, your miraculous outcome will be the only version that lives inside the Temple of Universes. The collapsing of the other two will become permanent. Over time, the Temple of Universes will change and evolve with you. It might look the same for a while, but don't be surprised when one day you find a different Temple of Universes waiting for you. As I write this, my Temple holds a beautiful bookcase filled with books that I've written in my future. My Temple holds my dreams of all the things I want to create. I find Bjarne inside there often, sitting on a couch smiling at all my creations. In a way, he's creating with me by observing my creations into reality. Our potential coexists with the people we lost.

Now we'll go into great detail about these three different realities so when the time comes for you to do this part of the journey you'll feel as though you've been there before, and your Survivor won't wig out. Remember, each week you add a new journey, until the whole Temple Journey is complete. Each journey goes deeper, so this is the deepest we've gone so far.

The Average Outcome Universe

Let's start by describing the Average version. The logical version of the future is the one that's extracted from the elements that make up our lives today. We tend to observe what our limited brain has already observed and experienced before. We stay in the same universe, the reality we know, because we don't dare leap outside it. So, given the elements that make up our lives, we can more or less guess how our life is going to look ten years from now. If everything continues in the same trajectory, the future will look a specific, predictable way. You'll live more or less in the same city. You might even live in the same house. You're possibly going to have the same core group of friends you have now. You might find a new partner. You might change jobs or your career or you might just stay where you are. This version is the logical future. If you had to guess, this is the way it would look. Throw in a few good things, some bad. A few surprises. Tie it with a bow. You're observing all these things and you're creating them from your observation. This is how any of these versions becomes a reality. Your brain generates a logical outcome from all the past patterns it has come across. I'm not saying there's anything wrong with a life lived in a status quo, but if you could have a life full of beautiful surprises, then why not observe that one?

The Survivor Universe

Inside the Temple, you'll also find the version of the universe reflecting your doubts and fears that the self creates. This version has the most chance of taking place because fear is an intense emotion and holds strong beliefs. It's almost as though we're being pulled toward worry, that the observation of our fears is a routine-based experience. We spend time observing our own fears daily. For the first three years after my loss, I spent every waking moment worrying about so many things. I know you've been there. This is a dangerous place to be.

In the upcoming journey, we're going to collapse the Survivor Universe (the version of your life based on worry and fear—for example, my worry-filled projection of running out of money so I couldn't buy health insurance for my girls—and the Average Outcome Universe—the logical version of your life explained above). I'll ask you to say no to them, unless you really like your life and don't want to change a thing, and that's fine. But have some fun with this journey. I know—fun with physics? Fun rebuilding and advancing our lives? Fun with our consciousness. Yes, yes, yes, and yes.

As I've said, to "collapse" a version of the universe is to remove that version. When you observe one possibility, it changes paths in the future. When a psychic or a prophet gives you a reading, that person gives you only one possibility. That's why I advise being cautious about psychics reading your future. If you observe the possibility that's predicted for you, and it's not a good one, and you believe the psychic is reading the future correctly, then this possibility can very well take place. So we're going to collapse these two versions—the Average Outcome Universe and the Survivor Universe—and focus on the universe we desire and observe in the Temple. Before we go any farther I want to share with you some examples from my students in class and what their experience was when they experienced the Temple of Universes for the first time.

The students in my class experienced such freedom during and after this journey. Three women who lost their husbands felt hugely liberated.

Claudia, who lost her beloved husband and who now lives with her beautiful daughter, said that collapsing the Survivor Universe "put me in charge of my life instead of allowing fear and worries to run it. One thing that I found very interesting is that it also allowed me to 'change' the past, or at least my perception of the past. So there were also the components of healing and forgiving that are so very important to me and my journey."

When Nancy, an amazing and strong woman and the mother of two incredible young adults, first collapsed the universe that didn't serve her anymore, said that it felt like "literally watching them shrink like an accordion." It was extremely powerful for her—that she could make them disappear.

When Carrie, who also lost her husband, collapsed the Survivor and Average realities, she said, "I felt an opening of possibilities— hope, really. I felt that expansion physically, and since then, I've been very conscious of collapsing my worries, and that has been life-changing. I'm working toward the life I want and see in the Temple!"

These women and others in the class were able to bring that feeling of liberation and ability to say no to anything that doesn't align with their miraculous universe, any Survivor worry, and yes to the opportunities that appear.

The Miraculous Universe

Imagine a life full of possibilities, love, adventure, and joy. This is what the Miraculous Universe reality is about. When we collapse the other two realties and focus on this one, we have a chance at rewriting our future. I want to share a story about one of my students, Laura. She had lost her husband a few years ago. During that time, she'd also lost financial security, and the journey back was really hard for her. When she spent time in the Temple of Universes, she felt that for the first time in her life she had the power to choose the outcomes of her own life. "The power to make a choice. It's been life-changing for me to know that I don't have to accept what some people have tried to make me believe about myself or how my life was going to go. For example friends would tell me things such as, 'You'll never own a home again.' Well, yes I will, and my name is now on the mortgage of our new home. 'You'll have to fly under the radar for the rest of your life.' Well, I don't feel that way at all anymore. I actually have a decent credit rating and have my name on a credit card again. To collapse all of that negativity—it's changed everything."

One of my students, Peter, lost his dad when he was four years old and he hadn't thought about him much since he started the class. His first journey to the Temple of Universes seemed to surprise him. His Temple appeared in the form of an old ramshackle house. "I recognized the place—it was this old beat-up house. I could have never guessed that's what it was going to be. I was looking for an actual Temple I had never seen before, maybe from somewhere new," Peter told me. "Somehow, I felt I'd been there before. The familiarity made it real for me, and that realness filled me with a sense of ease. My brain seemed able to trust this place."

"Was there anyone there with you?" I asked.

"Yes. A man. I feel he's my Super Watcher."

"How do you know?"

"I don't know, but I felt this very strange connection. As if I'd known this man before, as well as I know myself. The journey was, let's say, vivid," Peter said, his eyes wide. "When you asked us to collapse (remove) the Survivor-based reality and focus on the miraculous reality, everything changed. Inside my Temple of Universes, the reality I kept was the one with my father before he passed. In that reality he is there guiding me and sharing with me how proud he is of all I've accomplished. I felt his presence strongly. I also saw my dog that I'd lost prior to my dad's passing. Even though this reality isn't something I could bring back, it felt good to visit. I returned with a feeling of joy I hadn't experienced in a while. In the Temple of Universes, as I was looking at this one reality, I also saw myself living in a high-rise overlooking the city. I was startled by that image. I guess I wasn't expecting it. I must have chosen it and that's why it came through."

"Yes, we all have multiple versions of what can happen in our lives," I said, "and it's scary to believe that we can actually make those unwanted versions come true."

"Okay," Peter said, then looked away. He seemed skeptical.

"What's the one thing you remember bringing back from this new reality you saw inside the Temple of Universes?" I ask.

"I don't know if it's any one thing as much as a feeling of . . . I guess a sense of belief that I can make this new life happen. Living in a high-rise building with such a beautiful view. I can't explain it, it felt as if I had certainty while inside the Temple of Universes, certainty I rarely have in my regular life. So that's what I'm going to try to carry with me," Peter said, a smile sneaking in, "that feeling, and the ability to see the possibilities."

The Miraculous Universe is the most miracle-filled life you can possibly imagine. The life of your wildest dreams coming true. When you witness this life, allow the expanded consciousness of the Temple World to show you the beauty of this life, and try to interfere as little as possible. And when you're there, look at everything and strive to be very detailed in your observations. If you're looking at your home, notice the bedsheets. Is there a pattern? What color are they? If you have plants in your home, what type are they? What shade of green are the leaves? Look at the view. What people are in your life? What's taking place? What are you wearing? Do you go somewhere during your day? What do you do every day? That's the version of life that you're going to go back to every day when you take this journey.

Every time you go into the Temple of Universes and observe this reality, look around, examine details. You may find new details each time. Observe them all, take them in.

Precise and detailed observation while inside the Temple is a necessity. At first it will be challenging to be precise, but the more you journey to the Temple, the more you will be able to notice. As you move forward in the journey, you'll feel the desire to observe more closely, to notice more detail—the fabric of the curtains inside your dream home; the way the couch is sitting against the wall; the air that comes in through the window; the smells emanating from your kitchen; the person there you don't recognize. The more detail you take in, the greater your immersion; and the greater your immersion, the easier it is to convert the energy of the Temple of Universes to the matter of our 3-D reality.

Every time you return from the journey to the Temple of Universes and are back here in 3-D reality, look for some of the images you saw while there, here in your life. For example, you might go to a friend's house and discover she has a new table that is similar to one that appeared inside your Temple of Universes. Or you might visit a new town and see a house there that looks just like the one you saw in your miraculous universe. These are not coincidences. Your brain is seeking to find in 3-D what you saw on your journey and often, just as with the object exercise, it will succeed.

There are infinite possible lives, infinite versions of this life. And all versions can exist. You now get to choose the one that is made of beautiful miracles. I look forward to your journey in this chapter. I truly can't wait to see what you collapse, what you keep, and what you bring with you in your 3-D life.

The Temple of Universes Journey

Find a comfortable chair in a quiet place where you won't be disturbed. Read the instructions once or twice before you close your eyes to take the journey. Remember to have something on hand—a notebook, an iPad, etc.—to record your experience after the journey. If you'd like, you can play the corresponding sound vibration or other music, or simply proceed in silence. Relax your shoulders. You're in a safe space.

Now we'll journey all the way to the Temple of Universes along the familiar pathway. This is a journey that builds on itself, so as always, we'll begin with the Door, cross its threshold, connect with your Super Watcher and, together, travel through the Portal. After traveling through the Portal and spending time with your loved one, however, you won't return immediately to this 3-D reality. This is the moment you'll instead discover your Temple.

1. You're now on the other side of the Portal, possibly where you found yourself last time or perhaps in an entirely new location. Notice who else is there with you. Is your beloved there? Does your beloved want to come with you? Do you want your loved one to come with you to the Temple? Or is there a message he or she wants to pass on to you now before you go to the Temple? If so, what's that message?

2. Once you're ready, look toward the horizon. You will see your Temple of Universes. Be open to however it appears. It will be unique to you. As you approach your Temple, observe what it looks like. Is it made of stone? Does it have pillars?

3. Enter your Temple. Once inside, pause and look around. On your first visit, you'll see it contains three distinct areas: the

Average Outcome Universe, the Survivor Universe, and the Miraculous Universe. The Average Outcome will be to your left, the Survivor to your right, and the Miraculous straight ahead.

4. First, head for the Average Outcome Universe. Go toward that space—maybe you open a door, walk through an archway, or just take a few steps to an open space. Once there, look at your life, observing from the place where you are now. See what the Average Outcome Universe looks like. It's neither bad nor good, just a logical version of the future given the beliefs you have about your life now. Look at your home in the future, your relationships, your work, your life. All the different aspects. Feel the feelings that come along with this life and just take it all in. Now walk away from that life. Soon you'll collapse it.

5. Gently walk into the life that is on the right side, your Survivor Outcome Universe. That life is made of your doubts, worries, and fears about what could go wrong. You're not going to spend much time here because you want to observe this universe as little as possible. You'll just walk out of that life, the life of worry, doubts, and fear, and say good-bye.

6. And now, at once, we're going to collapse those two lives, the Average Outcome life and the Survivor Outcome life. We're going to decide that those are not our lives. We are not going to think about them or observe them moving forward. We

collapse them now. Both at once. It's more powerful that way. And just like that, they're collapsed.

7. You're now standing in the entranceway. Look directly in front of you to the place in the Temple that awaits you, that's been awaiting you. You move in a straight line to it. This place is so beautiful. It holds the most incredible life for you; it pulses with joy. As you walk toward that life, you see that you have everything you've ever wanted. You have the perfect people with you. You have work that you love. This version of your life, this version full of miracles, is the one that you choose to exist in. You wake up every day in your 3-D life saying, "I can't believe I get to live this life. It's amazing and it's beautiful." Know that every day, when you return to the Temple and observe this life, more of this life will be revealed.

8. Walk out of the Temple. As you're moving away from the Temple, turn back one last time and say good-bye for now and know that this is your special place of creation. This is where you go to pray, to create, to see what's in your future. It's where everything lives before it comes into physicality here in this 3-D reality.

9. As you walk away, you see the Portal waiting for you. Jump right in and take the journey back at the speed of light. All the way. Through the galaxies and the stars, this incredible beautiful cosmos we live in, out the other side.

10. Walk toward your Door.

11. Now pass through your Door, feeling the energy of this space with all the goodness that it brings you. This time you've brought with you a glimpse of your new life. Take a deep breath. In and out. We're back.

Was This All My Imagination?

Now you're back from your Temple Journey and you may be wondering, *Was it real? Did I really see my future? Was there an actual Temple? Did I collapse all the unwanted things in my life? Could it be this easy?* Unfortunately, it's not quite that easy. As we mentioned earlier, your Survivor will fight to hold on to the fear-based life. To hold on to the fears and doubts. Your brain will spend the next few hours hijacking this experience. Your old beliefs will come in and say things such as, *that was just your imagination, nothing more.* You'll forget about the multiverse. You'll dismiss the observer-effect theory.

But I beg you to do something very important before this begins to happen. Share your experience with someone in your book club, if you are reading this book with a group, with a friend who is open-minded, and share as soon as possible. Recall your experience and describe out loud to another person the details you saw in the Temple. Write them down. Find pictures that mirror what you saw and put them on your fridge, on your phone. Interrupt the hijacking for as long as possible. Ultimately, in the first few weeks—the week you take the journey daily and the few that follow—your brain will keep on winning. It will keep on telling you it was all an illusion, a figment of your imagination.

But it wasn't. It isn't. And what you see and experience isn't "just your imagination." It's the vision of your infinite cosmic consciousness. Alan W. Watts tells it like it is. And when I think of him I know that even though he may not have spoken of the Temple, he lived his life from a place of awareness and consciousness. This comment of his has stayed with me:

> *You have seen that the universe is at root a magical illusion and a fabulous game, and that there is no separate "you" to get something out of it, as if life were a bank to be robbed. The only real "you" is the one that comes and goes, manifests and withdraws itself eternally in and as every conscious being. For "you" is the universe looking at itself from billions of points of view, points that come and go so that the vision is forever new.* [5]

Billions of points of view, points that come and go. You saw your life from a very different point of view that can stay or go. Your brain will send it away, and this is why I'm asking you to bring forth your memory of the journey and replay it over and over again. And every day go back there to see more miracles and possibilities and to observe them like a kid riding with no training wheels or spotting the Big Dipper for the first time. In awe.

Your experience of the Temple of Universes fundamentally allows you to observe your consciousness and make it into matter.

Just because we shut down the 3-D reality while we journey into the Temple, it doesn't mean that we remove ourselves from that reality, it just means that we can understand it better. We begin to understand that this 3-D reality is only a small part of the bigger picture. This day-to-day reality is always our foundation and we will always come back to it. But our reality has its roots in something grander, outside the linear thinking that takes place here. Also, our beloveds are part of that greater reality. They just don't appear to be part of the 3-D world. Just like the Temple can't be seen. Just as the other dimensions can't be seen. Just as dark matter can't be seen. They all exist, but not in the way we experience in the third dimension.

You might be asking, "What are we really doing here in this book? Is this a feel-good book, glossing over the tragedy of losing my beloved and the mess I'm left with called life? How is this fake journey helping me pay the bills, sleep alone at night when I'm scared to death and missing his embrace? How is it at all helping with the reality of this life?"

Gradually, the Temple is reminding you who you are, that death and birth are not real but just what our consciousness brings to light. Don't cling to the illusion because it's easy to believe. Cling to the miracles that await you. Cling until your fingers can't anymore, and when you find yourself on the edge of your mind, outside the regular paths, beyond the perceived limitations, and believing for the first time that the Temple is a real location where your potential lives—then anything is possible. Accepting the nature of our universe as a mystical place and allowing that mysticism to come along with us on this journey is the first step to shedding the beliefs that keep us hostages to the same patterns and sequences, as if we were numbers in a formula or letters in the alphabet.

You are the entire formula, the alphabet. You are everything there is. Everything there will ever be. If you're unable to accept your Super Watcher, your higher self that is deeply aware of the laws of the universe, and creates and observes, you're denying your own existence. Without your cooperation the Super Watcher cannot evolve. And even though the Temple Journey at this point may be a stretch for your brain, it's actually one step closer to where we're ultimately going.

As we move deeper into the journey, you'll find that you'll begin letting go of your attachment to your beloved. But you'll gain a sense of them in your life, guiding you. I want to share an insightful conversation I had with one of my class participants. As you will read there is a lot of letting go that is taking place because of the Temple Journey. Surrendering to what the new life brings without guilt.

Louisa lost her husband a few years ago and couldn't see him during the first couple of times doing the Temple of Universes Journey. She had seen him in the earlier journeys prior to the Temple of Universes. Then on the third journey, to her surprise there he was. "He was kind of standing back," she told the class, "smiling, happy watching me and the kids in this new home in the Temple of Universes. It was beautiful. So much light streaming through the windows. The kids were laughing and playing. By his presence, and his distance, it felt as if he was happy about how are lives were going. Then he left and I stayed. And that was fine. I was happy.

"When you said, 'Time to come back,' my first thought was, *I don't want to go back.* The feeling was so amazing there. Yet, at the same time, I've been at such peace all week knowing this life I've seen is possible. To have the approval from my husband was a really big moment for me. I felt it because even before he died, he told me that he wanted me to be happy and to find love again. I have felt guilt about remarrying but to be in that space and to see that he was so supportive of it were very validating and freeing."

Your Homework for This Week

Once you start seeing your miraculous life emerging inside—and outside—the Temple, don't be surprised if your Survivor raises its voice louder than ever before. It doesn't like it when you change things and take chances. How do you quiet your Survivor? Learn to see yourself as a creator. Someone created from the cosmos, who is capable of creating miracles, of creating universes. Because you are. You are more powerful than your body can ever be. Intelligent beyond the limits of your brain. You are a creator—a god, the universe itself, the force behind the making of your life.

It is hard to accept, to truly believe, that we are the universe witnessing itself, the miracle creating miracles, the player playing the game we invented. But we are. We don't have to fear our 3-D reality. Even though we can't escape the human condition altogether, we can open the Door to another dimension where our consciousness will continue to live on forever. Even in our human form, we all have the power to access this timeless existence within the Temple World. Go there and find the God you were born to be.

the temple mirror

You must first have the knowledge of your power;
second, the courage to dare; third, the faith to do.

—CHARLES F. HAANEL[1]

When I looked in the Mirror inside the Temple, I saw myself at a beach in Cancun that my husband, David, and I went to many times," Maria told the class. She seemed light, happy. Her eyes shone and she was smiling. "When I saw myself on the beach," she said, "to my surprise, I had really short hair. The last time I wore hair that short I was much younger. I never liked my hair short, but in the mirror, there it was.

"I also looked much thinner in the Mirror, healthier," Maria said, "not that I'm big *now*, but you know what I mean. And one more thing. I was holding a baby sea turtle, this tiny, tiny little turtle. Isn't that strange? I was with a group on the beach, and we all had these baby sea turtles. I'm not sure why.

"So there I was on the beach. I had very short hair. I was very thin. I was very healthy. And I had a baby sea turtle," Maria said happily. "Then we set the turtles in the water and watched them swim out into the ocean."

"What year was it, the year that you last had short hair?" I asked.

"I think it was probably in 2000."

"What was happening in 2000?" I asked.

"I don't know," Maria said. "I'll have to think about it."

"Yes, I think the short hair is meaningful. I wonder what the message is."

"Okay." Maria picked up her pen and notepad. "I'm writing down these questions. I have to write everything down," Maria said, smiling.

"I understand that! Now, about the baby turtle, since you mentioned how healthy you looked, what has it to do with your health?"

Maria added that question to her list of questions, some of which she can ask when she returns to the Temple on her next journey. Then she looked up. "Rebirthing my health. It was a baby, and it was being released into the ocean. So, the ocean of my consciousness." Maria scribbled more notes on her pad.

"Also, I kept seeing a man, but I was not focusing on the man. I was focusing on my health," Maria added.

"He can be there, too," I said. "He might be part of your health journey. One of the things I hear a lot lately is that when someone's close to accomplishing something, receiving good news, or drawing near to something great, they say, 'Let's not talk about; I don't want to jinx it. I don't want to be disappointed.' We are taught not to think about something good just in case it doesn't happen, but we should be doing the opposite. We should observe the version of the reality we want rather than avoid seeing it so we won't be disappointed if it doesn't happen. So if there's a man next to you while you're feeling healthy, why not?"

"Okay, I'll take it," Maria said and laughed quietly.

What Maria saw in the Mirror in her Temple was quite unexpected, but that is how The Mirror works. You never know what you will see and how it will make you feel. How it will impact your life. The Mirror Journey can be a transformative experience. You'll be taking that journey in a little while, and I can't wait for you to experience the Mirror and see your own message in it. But first let me explain to you how it is possible to receive such an important message in a Mirror inside your consciousness.

What Will You Experience?

You might think that after collapsing the Average Outcome and Survivor Universes and bringing into reality the Miraculous Universe, your time in the Temple would be done—and that your next journey would take you elsewhere. But the next journey takes place *within* the Temple. There is something within the Temple that is vital to your greater journey. What is it? A Mirror. Yes, an actual Mirror. Just like the one you have in your bathroom or bedroom. Situated simply on a wall or on a dresser. In my Temple, the Mirror is always on a wall. The size of the Temple Mirror is different for everyone. It might be huge or it might be as small as a hand mirror, just big enough for you to see your image. You must be wondering, what I am to do with a Mirror inside the Temple of Universes? You look in it. And as you do you will see yourself not as you've always seen yourself in 3-D reality, but in ways you were not expecting. Be open to what will be there for you.

The Temple Mirror is almost like the glue of yourself, the glue that restores wholeness to the infinite pieces that make you. It is not that these pieces were ever separate from you, but it is that you have not been guided to look for them. A whole *you* is reflected within this Mirror, for everything that you are missing is there. And everything that you think you never had comes back to you. For example, if you're experiencing loneliness in your day-to-day life, you might see yourself with a group of people inside this reflection, as there is part of you that is not lonely and has never been lonely. And that part of you is part of the loneliness you are feeling. Once these two seemingly separated parts come back together, the whole self feels no lack of anything. My class participants would often see someone they'd never seen before inside their Mirror. Quite a few of them saw someone standing behind them. If the Mirror represents the whole, then you may see your beloved there also and you may see someone you are about to meet.

The Mirror is just like everything else inside the Temple Journey: without time and space, and nonlocal. Whatever is missing or seems lacking in your life you will find in the Temple Mirror. Just like you would if you were able to see the unbroken wholeness in a tangible, visible way. I also want to mention that if there has been a shadow in your past, something unresolved, you might see things that will help you understand your past better. Sometimes it will feel hard to look in the Mirror because you may see a part of you that you have been avoiding. The Mirror will gather everything in its reflection. So when you stand in front of it, you might feel a little afraid to look in. Don't be. Stand tall, arms at your side, open to everything that will be shown to you. Take it all in, knowing that the Mirror has chosen the image from a pool of infinite possibilities to reflect back to you. You might even see your beloved looking in the Mirror with you as though supporting you, providing gentle guidance.

We Are Part of the Whole

As I mentioned earlier, the Temple Mirror is not bound by gravity, time, or space. The Temple Mirror isn't influenced by the rules of a 3-D world. It's not fragmented into the "I" and the "it." When you look inside the Temple Mirror, you remember that you belong everywhere. You are the Temple World. You are the Super Watcher. You are the Temple of Universes. And you are the people you lost. We are never separate from them. Your whole includes all the people you love and have loved. As we discussed in the beginning of the book, we step into the Temple World having guided our brain to exit the 3-D experience and enter a world where there is no loss, no end of time. A place where we never stop existing.

Just like the Temple World, there is nothing linear about what the Mirror reflects. What it shows you comes through from a place of connection rather than separation, which is what we are used to in our 3-D life. The Temple Mirror connects you to the wholeness of yourself. David Bohn, one of the most significant theoretical physicists of the twentieth century, wrote about what he called the holistic principle of undivided wholeness, which he described as the "unbroken wholeness of the totality of existence as an undivided flowing movement without borders."[2] I thought about what he meant by this and how it would translate in the world of the Temple. Bohn believed that there is a deeper reality, an ocean of energy floating around us that is intangible. Everything is interconnected and is moving at the same time. Everything is inside everything else. The Mirror inside the Temple is our way of experiencing the whole Bohn describes. Experiencing the whole inside a smaller space, in an actual mirror. There is no here or there; everything is always connected. This is why our observations in our 3-D world aren't pure. We can only see the world around us as divided.

The Mirror Journey ignites the *Wholeness Experience*. Bohn wrote that "thought itself is a process of movement and that thought may be a part of reality as a whole."[3] Your thoughts in front of the Mirror originate from your whole self. In front of the Mirror, your observations are not easily influenced by your 3-D thinking patterns, patterns that result from a lifetime of conventional knowledge. In front of the Mirror you get to glimpse a new narrative for yourself. To see your soul from a vantage point that has been forgotten, left behind, maybe even erased from your memory in this life. The Temple Mirror isn't influenced by the rules of a 3-D world. There is no end there, no loss of memory of a past existence.

The Mirror holds all of it together, and when we stand there it reveals the whole we need to see. You are about to see yourself in ways that have never been possible before because your perception of yourself was made of a limited construct of reality.

One of the times I looked in the Mirror, I looked past my reflection and saw that behind myself, hung a series of large paintings. The paintings were beautiful, bold, and vibrant. But instead of feeling joy, I panicked. I turned away from the Mirror and immediately searched inside the Temple for the books I had written. I realized then that I feared my dreams of making art. This insight blew me away. I had no idea that was a worry I had. I recognized in that moment that I had been avoiding painting out of fear that my books wouldn't be written. Part of the process of becoming whole, of course, is being able to come up against fear and limiting beliefs in a safe environment. With the expanded consciousness you experience in the Temple, you can look at your fears and limiting beliefs and let them go, transform them. The good news is the realizations come quickly and so does the shift from fear or panic to resolution and peace.

I then saw bookshelves with many copies of each of my books, all while the paintings were still hanging on the walls of my Temple in my Mirror. My reflection in the Temple Mirror suddenly appeared far more laid-back. Relaxed. Without worries. I was smiling. The Mirror brought forth wholeness. Where both dreams could be a part of my life. Without sacrifice. The painter reality started to become a reality. I now have paintbrushes in my office and at least three large canvases I've painted on. I now choose my paintings the same way I choose my books in my 3-D life.

We Are Nonlocal

When I first looked in the Mirror I was able to see what I could not see in the physical world, a version of myself outside my current beliefs and thoughts. A part of me that I had all but forgotten existed, but a part of me that had been there along. But where had it been if it hadn't been with me all this time? What if our lives are not where we think they are? What if they are not situated in one specific place? It appears that nothing is local. We are not stuck in one place, living out our routines, walking back and forth at the same spot. Instead, we are everywhere. Instead, once we interact with something or someone we are permanently entangled with them as if we keep interacting. Even though we don't seem to be. Nonlocality points toward a universe that knows no location, no separation, and no individuality. As explained in *The Physics of the Universe:*

> *Nonlocality suggests that the "separate" parts of the universe are actually potentially connected in an intimate and immediate way. Nonlocality is based in entanglement theory, where particles that interact with each other become permanently correlated, or dependent on each other's states and properties, to the extent that they effectively lose their individuality and, in many ways, behave as a single entity, even if, for example, they're on the other sides of the universe.*[4]

What if that were true? What if you are connected with everyone else, a part of a bigger whole existing everywhere and not just right here at your house? Your home and my home may be one and the same. Death and life, one and the same. Situated inside an entanglement with everything and everyone you have ever known.

In my Temple Journey class, the participants came from and lived in many parts of the world, yet when they went inside the

Temple World they experienced the journey together, as if they lived right next to each other.

In an article for *Scientific American*, George Musser gave a perfect example of nonlocality:

> *Physics experiments can bind the fate of two particles together so that they behave like a pair of magic coins. If you flip them, each will land on heads or tails—but always on the same side as its partner. They act in a coordinated way even though no force passes through the space between them. Those particles might zip off to opposite sides of the universe, and still they act in unison. The particles violate locality—they transcend space.*[5]

Location is not what we think it is. Just like time. It is an illusion. We are nonlocal beings and are in many ways scattered across the universe outside of time and space. The Mirror shows you your nonlocal self. It reminds you of your wholeness, that you belong not only to your life and your home but also to everything else—however far it is from you, however outside of time and space it appears. You are the Universe at a glance. You are a time traveler. You belong to more people than you imagined, and you occupy every dimension that we know exists. The purpose of the Temple Mirror is to reflect back to you that whole reality that includes all versions of your selves—past, present, future, possible. Wholeness in a nonlocal world means our seemingly fragmented selves are part of a whole that encompasses infinity in parallel lives. The Mirror within the Temple of Universes brings back the wholeness of the self to prove the nonlocal nature of our existence. Each part of us was not left behind in some other time of place, just like the people we lost are not trapped in the past tense. They can't be. They are with us, just like our whole selves never left us.

The Temple Mirror Effect

The Temple Mirror brings forth a self based on a journey of true wholeness, one that bypasses your losses, your problems, and allows you to observe yourself through a filter connecting everything you thought was separate within yourself. The Mirror can change the way you identify with your life and your life's events. Imagine that every time you go to the Temple Mirror and objectively observe what's there, and, when you return, you consciously choose to live your life from that whole self, everything in your life could change. For example, if you are in a troubled relationship and you interact with that person from the way the Mirror made you feel, then that troubled relationship is either going to be better or you will walk away from it.

But remember, as with any change, your Survivor is going to do everything possible to scare you back into your comfort zone. Especially if you're planning on creating the miraculous life you are seeing inside your Temple, and most important, bringing forth the beautiful person you see in the Mirror. The Survivor will have a hard time with your seeing your wholeness and your full power. And above all, with your believing in a much bigger vision for your life than the one your Survivor is allowing you to see. You are training your mind not to see the Survivor-made universe.

Our thoughts spring from our primal brain and our hard-wired programming for survival. We're not taught to believe we are whole, which is why, if we don't actively step in and reclaim our wholeness, our Survivors will completely run the show. Our Survivors could very easily continue dictating what we see, how we see it, how we feel about it, and what we do about it in our 3-D reality.

You need to be kind to yourself through this journey, reach out to those in your Temple Circle, visit your Temple daily to build your sense of faith, trust, comfort, and joy of possibility. If we can only select what best serves our higher self, our Super Watcher, then we create a different reality. Ultimately our goal is to consciously create a reality in which we feel in abundance and wholeness. The Mirror gets us closer to that goal by reminding us of our wholeness, of our nonlocality. And if we succeed in creating that reality, we will never find ourselves lost for long. Rejections will still take place, but less frequently. And while loss is unavoidable, it will be far less devastating, and we'll remain connected to our loved ones, still communicating with those who have transitioned to another dimension. I'm not asking for the creation of heaven on Earth, I am asking for the possibility of using our free will to create our own freedom from circumstances, which would be pretty close to heaven, I think!

In an interview in *The Atlantic*, cognitive scientist Donald Hoffman said, "Evolution shapes acceptable solutions, not optimal ones."[6] In other words, our ways of understanding our world derive from survival and self-protection. We have to find a way to break the code that has been operating for many thousands of years through our evolution. Somehow we can all find our way to a new code. A code of wholeness. The code I built is the Temple World, where we consciously choose to have thriving experiences even if we are scared to have them at first. The more we journey, the less fear will be part of our 3-D lives.

The Fifth Mode of Prayer

Across cultures and time, people have used prayer to cope with fear and find hope. In many ways, the Temple World is a big prayer. A nonlocal church. One that goes where you go. And is always a part of you. You see, thousands of years ago, people were taught how to pray. From these ancient practices, prayer researchers have defined four overarching modes of prayer: (1) colloquial, or informal; (2) petitionary; (3) ritualistic; and (4) meditative. These four forms all involve speaking to the divine, listening to the divine, and contemplating the divine. In his book *Secrets of the Lost Form of Prayer*, Gregg Braden writes of a fifth mode of prayer, the "lost mode," a mode of praying without words. In the fifth mode of prayer, we get lost in the feeling of the prayer, immersing ourselves in the joy and peace we'll experience when our prayer has been answered. This collapses the time between the asking and the answering, focusing on the gratitude and appreciation that fill our souls.[7]

In this kind of prayer, we aren't asking for help from the divine source; we feel as if the prayer has already been granted, so there's no need to ask. This is the feeling you get inside the Temple World, Braden's fifth mode of prayer. We go inside a place away from fear and grief that vibrates with the feeling of love and peace. There's no feeling of helplessness there, just knowing that everything is as it should be. We are able, through this feeling of love, to communicate with divine intelligence. And when we do, we heal.

I want to share my own story about this feeling and my subsequent evolution into a whole self that is nonlocal and lives inside the Mirror, which has been completely unexpected. Never in my wildest dreams would I have anticipated this massive change in my life. My experience shows how this feeling of wholeness and deep knowing of self can be entirely life-changing. And, for the record, I'm going to repeat what I've said before: your brain does not know the difference between what it sees in your mind and what it sees in this 3-D reality. And when your brain becomes comfortable with a new vision, the new experience, it brings more of it to your everyday reality. Just as you brought all the objects after you went through the Door, just as it brings synchronicity, it will bring to life what you have seen inside the Temple World.

The Strides That Changed My Life

In my first journeys into the Temple World, I moved slowly, timidly, because I didn't know what to expect. But after traveling to the Temple World for a few weeks, I became bolder, I began walking through the Door, holding myself taller and taking bigger strides.

The image of myself I started to see in the Mirror deepened the changes I was feeling in the way I carried myself and moved in the Temple World. I saw a stronger, more fit, younger self. This image grew clearer with every visit. These changes affected how I felt inside and how I saw the world. There were moments when I felt the way I did when I was twenty years old. My linear concept of time started to collapse and was replaced with an entirely new experience. I felt ageless and timeless. I could tell I was younger but not in a way I'd ever been. It was a different me who was stepping forward, one I hadn't experienced on this Earth.

The biggest transformation was the gliding experience. I glided gracefully like Daenerys Targaryen, Mother of Dragons, from *Game of Thrones,* and my strides were long, powerful, and purposeful. On each visit to the Temple World, the path to the Door was no longer flat, as it had been previously, but a steep hill that I bounded up with ease. My new stride changed the way I felt about my body. Suddenly the gliding and striding sensation from the Temple World appeared in my 3-D life.

The gliding feeling would last about a day, wearing off unless I took another journey through the Door. Each time I went in, this renewed version of me was faster and stronger, and each time I returned, I was stunned to find my body taking on the stronger physical presence of my Temple self.

I knew that I could bring back an object from the Temple World, but this was different. I wasn't just bringing into this reality an object from beyond the Door, I was bringing back an altered *me*. During that first week when this empowered version of myself appeared in the Mirror, I started eating less, and I lost a couple of pounds. My food cravings diminished in both intensity and frequency, and I started to move my body more.

During the weeks that followed, I watched that woman returning from the Temple World, running like a warrior through the Door back to this reality. Without consciously choosing to do so, I started to look for things in my life that would help me to lose weight and increase my strength. I suddenly had much more interest in these areas—exercise and food choices—than I'd had before. I signed up with a trainer at my local gym. I found a doctor who would weigh me every week and hold me accountable. As I'm writing this chapter I've let go of twenty pounds. I'm physically stronger, and I feel more and more like the warrior woman of my Temple Journeys.

I started writing this book to help people find the loved ones we lost and I stumbled upon a better life. I stumbled upon the universe that holds my beloved husband but also my wholeness. The parts of me that I didn't know where missing.

What Will You Observe?

The very first time I looked in the Mirror, time collapsed, taking me to a place I'd forgotten existed. I saw myself as an ancient woman who'd lived many lives on the Earth plane. My hair was long and my clothes appeared to be from another time, an ancient time. Behind me, I saw a large library of books. I'd written all of them. I immediately recognized this version of my life and of myself. This was a person I'd known all my life. Within the Mirror I saw all the versions of myself that had been and that could be.

It was as though I held a mirror in front of my soul and could at last see all the things I'd always wanted to see and discover all the things I'd always wanted to know. I saw my soul's journey, unified in greater experience and encompassing all lives and possibilities. Yet I was restricted to this one 3-D reality I lived in. Inside the Mirror, I observed the truth about all my potential lives. I could see my purpose here more clearly. I now had so much more certainty about what I was here in this life to do. It was as though I were being shown memories that would align with the woman warrior powerfully running through the entryway at the beginning and the end of the journey. I saw her in the Mirror in all her glory. In all my glory. The woman inside the Mirror was me.

About that time, I came across these words: "If you bring forth what is within you, what you bring forth will save you. If you do not bring forth what is within you, what you do not bring forth will destroy you" (Didymos Judas Thomas to Jesus Christ, Gospel of Thomas 70). Destruction for you and me means living a life that is not whole and complete if we don't know all parts of ourselves. The Mirror doesn't show us a future life or a past life as if they are separate from us; it shows us what we're ready to see— aspects of our souls that have always been there. Our past lives and our future lives are not separate from us because everything is connected and time doesn't exist inside the Temple. And as I said, in the Temple World, all these aspects are far easier to deal with, on our way to healing and realizing all we're capable of, being our whole selves, living our miraculous lives.

You can collapse Survivor and Average Outcome Universes to see your ideal life, the Miraculous Universe the Temple is showing you, but feeling like the person who could have this life is different altogether. The Mirror represents the you who could have this life.

It allows you to see your soul in ways that are impossible by any other method.

The Mirror also allows you to observe yourself in ways that may initially create conflict and duality within you—the duality of how you see yourself outside of the Temple World verses inside the Temple World.

I once saw myself in the Mirror dressed as a Japanese empress. I was confused and thrown by that, as I have never been to Japan and don't know anything about Japanese history and culture. I decided to investigate the history of Japan and its people. What I learned empowered my life. This Japanese empress from my reflection began influencing the perception I had of myself. I felt as if I was more powerful than ever before. Another student saw herself hanging upside down but felt joy from it. She was going through so much change in her life that the image of herself upside down made a lot of sense. Her hair was also sticking out as if an energy jolt was going through it. She laughed out loud when she saw herself like this. It reminded her also to find the humor in all of the change that was taken place.

What you see in the Mirror is completely unexpected. Don't try to imagine, control, or predict it. This is the beauty of the Temple World, after all; it has its own intelligence, it's inside the divinity of the cosmos, and it's part of you.

The Mirror Journey

Being one with the cosmos is hardly a new idea. The ancient words "as above, so below, as within, so without, as the universe, so the soul," attributed to Hermes Trismegistus, purported author of the sacred Hermetic corpus, have always resonated deeply with me. Modern science has made many discoveries in the past few years that seem to support this view of undivided wholeness. We're finally realizing, increasingly, that we're one and the same with the cosmos. As inside the Temple, so outside the Temple. As in the Mirror, so in life.

Teachings that express this concept of wholeness claim it's impossible to study the universe without studying human beings. Conversely, it's impossible to study human beings without studying the universe. In his book *In Search of the Miraculous: Fragments from an Unknown Teaching*, Russian philosopher P. D. Ouspensky wrote of his time spent with twentieth-century spiritual teacher George Gurdjieff, who stated the impossibility of studying one without the other, then went on to say:

> *Man is an image of the world. He was created by the same laws which created the whole of the world. By knowing and understanding himself he will know and understand the whole world, all the laws that create and govern the world. By simultaneously studying the world and the laws that govern the world he will learn and understand the laws that govern himself. In this connection, some laws are understood and assimilated more easily by studying the objective world, while others can only understand through studying himself. The study of the world and the study of man must therefore run parallel, one assisting and furthering the other.*[8]

Human beings are far easier to observe than a microscopic atom or a telescopic galaxy. And yet, in the 3-D world, the illusion of separation means we are blind to our wholeness, to our true selves. Thus, to gain self-knowledge, I suggest that we must often look outside ourselves to see ourselves. Indeed, "as above, so below" goes hand in hand with another ancient adage, "know thyself." The Mirror gives us that ability.

Find a comfortable chair in a quiet place where you won't be disturbed. Read the instructions once or twice before you close your eyes to take the journey. Remember to have something on hand—a notebook, an iPad, etc.—to record your experience after the journey. If you'd like, you can play the corresponding sound vibration or other music, or simply proceed in silence. Relax your shoulders. You're in a safe space.

Now we'll journey all the way to the Temple of Universes, along the familiar pathway. This is a journey that builds on itself, so as always we'll begin with the Door, cross its threshold, connect with your Super Watcher, and together travel through the Portal and to your Temple.

1. When you get to the Temple of Universes, set an intention and focus on one area of your life that you want to improve. It could be health. It could be love. It could be wealth. Anything. Then move straight toward the Miraculous Universe that you've visited before. Now, what do you see? Remember, this life is the most incredible, fulfilling life you can imagine. What does that look like? Look at the details, the colors, the shapes, the people, the relationships.

2. Now it is time to find the Temple Mirror. It won't take long to locate it. It is most likely right there in front of you. It's beautiful. Once you spot it, look in the Mirror and take yourself in, the way you look in this reality inside the Temple of Universes.

3. What's different? What's there that you haven't seen before? Look at all parts of you—your chin, your eyes, your hair, your body and clothing, your energy, how you move. Also, how do you feel? What is different about how you feel? You realize there's something in the Temple, something you didn't know before, but the you reflected in the Mirror knows.

4. Make a point of remembering a few aspects of yourself in the Mirror that you want to appear in your 3-D life at home. Look in the Mirror one more time—take in the smile, the whole self. And the new feeling with you.

5. We're ready to leave the Temple. With your Super Watcher alongside you, walk toward your Portal. You go through the Portal at the speed of light in the midst of galaxies and stars. It feels incredible. You arrive at the other side of the Portal.

6. You see your Door and walk toward it. Holding in your mind all of the things that you saw and felt when you looked in the Mirror, cross back through the Door.

7. Take a deep breath and slowly come back here.

8. Open your eyes. Take a few minutes to record your journey, your objects, and the aspects of yourself you brought back with you.

Your Homework for This Week

The Mirror Journey is a profound one and life changing. But remember, we are journeying every day, and your experience will deepen and broaden as you spend more time in front of the Mirror. Soon those aspects of yourself you brought back with you will begin to show up in your life. From now on, during each journey you take to the Temple, focus on a specific aspect of your life. It could be health, wealth, love, or anything you want it to be. I prefer to be very specific when I'm standing before the Temple Mirror. With a clear intention, I am able to observe more clearly, which lends a hand in taking all that I have experienced in the Temple World into my 3-D world.

Every day this week go and look at yourself in the Mirror inside your Temple of Universes, then find your way to the Miraculous Universe you spent time in last week. And make sure you spend time there with the person you see in the Mirror; it might amplify your experience further. Share everything with a friend, a family member, and, of course, if you're in a Temple Circle, then do so there. Make sure you're writing everything down as well. Tap into the new feelings you experienced and the new person you felt like you were in the Mirror and do your daily activities from there. Speak from that personality. That newfound confidence. Tap into that identity, that persona you saw in the Mirror.

7

the field

Behind it all, is surely an idea so simple, so beautiful,
so compelling that when in a decade, a century or a millennium
we grasp it, we will say to each other, how could it have been
otherwise? How could we have been so stupid for so long?
—JOHN ARCHIBALD WHEELER

Dinea's face filled the screen during our virtual class. Her eyes shone as she described her experience on the journey to the Field—the final journey in the Temple World, which we've just completed.

"I was wearing a light blue, very ethereal, shimmery dress," Dinea said. "Outside the Temple, I was sort of float-walking into the Field. My Field was filled with beautiful wildflowers. The ground was silky, velvety like sand, but not as granular. Gorgeous butterflies were flying everywhere. There was a very light breeze flowing through beautiful rays of sunshine. Then I got to the part where we visited our 3-D world from inside the Field, where we looked at ourselves in our chairs, eyes closed, taking the journey. The me in the chair wasn't wearing the beautiful blue dress, but the clothes I'm wearing now, and the clothes glowed. I glowed.

And I looked at myself and said out loud to no one, 'Wow, I'm really beautiful.' I hadn't felt that way in a long time. I walked around that house. It was the house I live in now, but it appeared that I'd done a lot to it. Made amazing changes to it. It was so beautiful.

"My kids were at school, but I looked in their rooms, at the pictures of them on the mantel, and I felt such love for them, for their beingness, beautiful inside and out. I walked outside and down my street. I live in a great neighborhood. I kind of floated to my office, where I see patients and take care of kids every day. Looking at myself from inside the Field, I saw myself differently. *Yeah, that's me*, I thought. *I'm a really amazing doctor.* I saw how much love I give to those kids I take care of every day, how much love I give to my own children, to my friends, even to the barista I say hi to every morning at Starbucks. He always remembers my crazy name and gets my coffee ready for me before I can even order. I saw how much love they give to me. Looking at my life from inside the Field, I saw that it's beautiful. I'm blessed. I have so much love to give and to keep giving. And then, after I walked back into the Temple and was walking out again, I saw a little key by the Door," Dinea said with joy. "That was my object!"

"A key," Dinea said. "A little brass key. The head of the key had a little heart on it. I just grabbed it and took it with me through the Door. So I'm pretty happy right now. That was a really cool experience. I didn't want it to end."

"I feel your joy and happiness, even the energy of the key. I wonder what the key is and what it means," I said. "I love how you saw your life as being so beautiful, saw such blessings, and found such joy in your home, the work you do every day. I love how you saw your own beauty. It's an incredible gift to see your life the way you did. I feel that you immersed yourself in feelings of joy, bliss, appreciation, and gratitude. It's incredible."

Dinea nodded enthusiastically. "Most of the time in my day-to-day life I feel like all I'm doing is working, working, working. Hard. Taking care of the kids, taking care of everybody else, and doing all the other things I need to do around the house, with the kids, in the world. Going into my life here through the Field allowed me to step back and see myself, that there's a lot more going on here that I take for granted or often don't pay much attention to. But this trip gave me a different perspective. I saw things. I saw myself in a life that actually has been working these past five years since I lost my husband. It's a good thing, and I'm excited, and you're right, I'm not going back, I'm moving forward." Dinea stopped and took a breath. "I need a dress." She laughed.

The Field brings us closer to seeing our life through the eyes of the Temple. And when we do, well then, everything changes here in this reality. I say this every time but this next journey is one of my favorites because of the energy you feel throughout. It has giddiness. Bliss. And a new way to feel about everything. Enjoy.

What Will You Experience?

I've been obsessed with the space between us, between our bodies and our chairs, tables, appliances, our things—this seeming nothingness—for as long as I can remember. I was incredibly curious about this space around us even before Bjarne's passing from this dimension. Then I discovered that the nothingness between me and him is the same as what you and I are made of: invisible energy. We are all part of a sea of energy. We still exchange energy with the people we lost, but that exchange doesn't look the same way it used to. Still, it's there. This chapter is dedicated to the space between us, to the energy that nothingness is made of, and how that energy interacts with the living and with those outside the third dimension whom we have wrongly named the dead.

In this journey, we'll explore the field of energy that extends indefinitely throughout space and connects us to the world beyond matter, to everything and everyone in it. Just like gravity, it's a very significant force we live inside of every single day. We interact with the currents and charges that take place within this Field. In this journey we'll view our 3-D life from the perspective of the Field. We'll witness ourselves from outside this 3-D dimension, from outside time—from eternity. From this perspective, you'll know what you need to do, be, and feel about yourself and about your life. This allows us to grow beyond what we currently believe is possible, enrich our lives, live with far less fear, and feel more connected to those who've left this dimension.

Because everyone and everything—visible and not—are connected in this Field, it also connects the Temple World with our 3-D world. So this journey, while not the *last* Temple Journey you'll ever take, is the final step to giving you the tools to interact with both worlds. After that, journeying becomes a daily practice of growth, expansion, and connection with the 95 percent of the universe we cannot see.

On this journey, we'll explore how the Field interacts with your mind and your thoughts. As we know by now, there is no nothing, no nowhere, and no empty space. So let's jump right in this place of seeming nothingness that has everything in it, including our interactions. And, of course, your person who no longer lives in the same dimension as you but is part of this Field that surrounds you.

Nothing Is Full of Everything

As far back as the fifth century BCE, a Greek philosopher named Leucippus brought forth the concept that matter is made up of indivisible atoms.[1] Every single day, we live in and interact with a Field of energy that cannot be seen with the naked eye. That energy is called Zero Point Energy, or the vacuum state, the lowest vibrational state of energy. We measure vibrational states by the heat of an area. The faster particles move, or the more "excited" they get, the higher the temperature they create. For years it was believed that when the temperature dropped to absolute zero degrees, which is the lowest possible temperature, equivalent to minus 459 degrees Fahrenheit, there would be no movement, no energy. However, when scientists measured this energy, they found that even at absolute zero, there was movement.

Although Zero Point Energy is vacuum throughout the universe, according to NASA it's not empty. Instead, it contains "energetic charged particles, governed by magnetic and electric fields, and it behaves unlike anything we experience on Earth. In regions laced with magnetic fields, such as the space environment

surrounding our planet, particles are waves and virtual particles."
These particles, tossed about by plasma waves, zip into and out
of our physical world.[2] Imagine that particles enter our physical
world seemingly out of nowhere. Imagine that they interact with
matter, with us. Could it be that everything is created from this
energy field that looks like nothingness to us?

You, I, and those in the next town over, the town five thousand miles over—we're all connected. Whatever one person thinks
and feels interacts with and participates in everyone else's reality.
This connective field of energy exists. And it's incredibly powerful. It just doesn't look like matter does. It doesn't look like your
chair, your table, your floor. It looks like empty space. But it's
incredibly powerful. John Wheeler and his friend, the well-known
theoretical physicist and Nobel Prize winner Richard Feynman,
calculated that—be ready for this—just one small cup of Zero
Point Energy contains enough power to boil all the oceans on the
planet.[3] One small cup.

That's what you're tapping into when you make the invisible
real, when you act on an idea, create an amazing dinner, bring together a group of people to create change. That's powerful energy.
That's what's humming around you on a quiet, star-filled summer
night. As you gently process this, I'm going to add one more finding. According to Einstein, there's more matter per cubic centime-
ter of Zero Point Energy than the total mass of the entire universe,
which explains why Zero Point Energy is so powerful. There's
matter, and a lot of it, in places that look—but definitely aren't—
empty. More matter than you can ever imagine. What this means
is that matter doesn't end where your kitchen table ends. Matter

doesn't end at all. And everything you see in this reality around you has been generated by this Zero Point Energy. By bringing our attention to (observing) the Field that is made of this very powerful energy and interacting with it we can create what we witness.

Matter is vibration, low vibration. Energy is higher vibration. We see matter as it vibrates at a lower energy. But we interact with both matter and nonsolid energy. Everything is information that interacts within that energy. Our minds and bodies read this information and convert it into reality. Matter. Life. Whatever you want to call it. Thoughts, memories, and feelings don't live inside our bodies. The body just translates the energy and converts it into reality. Einstein's famous equation from 1905 $E=mc^2$ demonstrates that energy (E) is equivalent with matter (mass m).

Now, if Einstein was right about this and matter is equivalent to energy, then we could take this one step farther and say that by using the observer effect theory we can make matter out of the energy that surrounds it. By observing, choosing, and cocreating mindfully with the energy that surrounds you. Always. It not only surrounds you, but it's also inside you, outside you. You're part of this. You're in it together. It's as if you finally know you have a dance partner, that you haven't been dancing alone. You've been dancing with the universe. This is not the secret of life, it is the essence of life. The essence of you. You were born from this Field and you will go back to this Field. The person you loved and is no longer here is part of the Field, which connects everything together at all times.

The Temple Journeys you've been taking have prepared you to enter the Field. By this point in the journey you've learned so much. You've learned that death isn't real, that time isn't real, and that your consciousness isn't just inside you—it's everywhere. You've learned that you can choose different futures for yourself if you want to, and that by observing these futures, selecting one, you can bring that future into your life. You've learned that the deeper you go inside your consciousness and away from the ego, your Survivor, the more feelings of bliss and peace you experience. Now, this final step—the Field Journey—will take you deeper into your existence and allow you to see the connections between you and everything else.

I'm hoping your experience on this next journey will allow you to get closer to believing that the experiences you've had so far weren't figments of your imagination but your real-life inter-actions with the universe. You now have the tools to stop your brain from taking away all these experiences you have given your-self through walking into the Temple World. Your Survivor will want to interrupt this sense of knowing a greater truth and this experiencing even more than ever before. You will be filled with doubts, but you'll also be filled with a deeper understanding of the universe and yourself. Taking a journey to the Temple World each day will build your confidence, deepen your belief, and increase your ability to resist the very real pull of the Survivor.

The Field

As I sit on my deck looking out at the mountains, the redwoods, and the wildflowers growing in my garden, I think about the Field, about how everything is connected within it. Directly across from me, two trees grow about twenty feet apart from each other. Knowing they're not actually separate, it's just that my eyes see them that way, makes me realize that I, too, am connected with the trees. And if that's true, what else am I connected to? What does this kind of connection mean for our lives, both at the everyday level and in the bigger picture? How might the truth of that connection influence our existence and our emotional experience of ourselves?

If the trees, the space between them, the deck where I sit, and the keyboard I'm typing on are all connected to me and we are all connected to each other in the Field, then this means that the Field isn't just something abstract, the Field is my life—is life itself. I'm inside it, connected to it, a part of the creator and the created. We're not separate from our creation of our life, and our creation isn't separate from us. We're connected to everything we see and don't see, hear and don't hear. Our thoughts, material things, feelings, life experiences are all part of the Field.

As I close my eyes and see the trees, I see the energy that connects them to each other. Maybe if I sit here every day, observing that energy and envisioning branches connecting the trees, the trees will grow faster, closing the seeming gap. After all, the space between these trees is just an energy system that accelerates and populates when consciousness (me) observes its growth. The Field makes us understand how everything is connected to everything else without exception. My mind observing matter, observing energy, creating a new illusion.

There's a way to understand the Field in your everyday life. When you feel that you have a good idea or you're feeling inspired and create something from that inspiration, that's when you're interacting with the Field. Maybe the great idea or surge of inspiration felt unexpected, out of the blue? That's your whole self interacting with the energy field around you. You were communicating with something invisible. Your ideas and inspirations want to be brought from thought to reality.

Here's another example. When you daydream about something you want—a vacation, a new home, a new relationship—and you see yourself inside this new reality or illusion, the observer in you creates that dream in the Field. The more you observe yourself in the reality you desire, the more you're interacting with the Field. The more your consciousness interacts with the particles of the Field, the more you can change the Field. In our 3-D reality, of course, we take action as well—we book the flight, call a Realtor, get out more. The beauty is that by observing the reality we want, things fall into place more easily—synchronicities occur, such as finding objects in this reality that we found in the Temple World.

During the Field Journey, you'll intentionally interact with that energy. What happens when you witness a miracle? You become aware of how this energy works—how miracles work. Although we work with this energy every day, we don't realize it. Instead, we think that our thoughts, inspirations, and manifestations are just business as usual. And when we have an unexpected idea or surge of inspiration, or when a delightfully unexpected but desirable event occurs in this reality, we call it a miracle or amazing luck. But it's not a miracle. It's how we're meant to create, live, and experience our consciousness. We're supposed to intentionally connect with its intelligence—work with this energy, tap into this greater consciousness.

If you knew that the Field holds you, that you are the Field, wouldn't it be easier to interact with it? Your thoughts, your emotions, your memories, your whole being is inside that Field. You're always interacting with the Field. Up to this point, you've most likely been creating your life accidentally, however—bad thoughts and good. So why not interact intentionally from now on and see what happens next?

In *The Field*, author Lynne McTaggart writes that for a long time, modern physicists were aware of this Field but had ignored its power. "In ignoring the effect of the Zero Point Field," she writes, "they'd eliminated the possibility of interconnectedness and obscured a scientific explanation for many kinds of miracles." She says that leaving the effect of the Zero Point Field out of their equations "was a little like subtracting God."[4] And we really don't ever want to subtract the spiritual, the miraculous, or the divine from any of this.

McTaggart argues that once we grasp the implications of all encompassing connection with the universe, we will be forced to redefine what it means to be human—to reimagine what we are capable of.

If we are in constant and instantaneous dialogue with our environment, if all the information from the cosmos flows through our pores at every moment, then our current notion of our human potential is only a glimmer of what it should be. If we're not separate, we can no longer think in terms of "winning" and "losing." We need to redefine what we designate as "me" and "not-me," and reform the way that we interact with other human beings, practice business, and view time and space. We have to reconsider how we choose and carry out our work, structure our communities, and bring up our children. We have to imagine another way to live.[5]

I love how McTaggart illuminates the ways in which coming to a true understanding of the Field can deeply transform every aspect of our lives. That is what the Temple Journey is ultimately all about—a radical transformation of not only our understanding of life and what we call death—but of our life here in this 3-D reality. Once you cross the threshold of your Door, enter the Temple World, meet your Super Watcher, visit your Temple, look in its Mirror and, finally, dance with the Field, the unseen will never be "invisible" to you again. And once that happens, your life will never be the same.

What we are doing in the Field Journey is making the energy that connects us all, and of which we are all a part, visible. We are giving our brains the ability to "see" it and thus *believe* in it. When you make the Field visible and interact with it by choice, your intuition, creativity, and comprehension will grow stronger, faster, clearer, more focused. Our interactions with the energy around us offer us a deeper understanding of and connection to ourselves and the greater world around us that we can't see. This is the difference between wishing for something better in our lives and asking to be shown how to improve that something and receiving a direct answer. No more accidental creation. Just a direct visible sense of manifestation that has always been there waiting for you.

What the Field Journey Is Really About

The Field is about the truth of who you are, which lives in your consciousness and transcends your body. It's everything that lies between this body and the person you lost. You're connected to the person you lost through the journey to the Temple World. In this journey, you'll realize that the empty space you seemingly see beyond yourself isn't empty at all. The Field actually holds the Temple World inside it, not the other way around. Why didn't I call this whole process the Field Journey? Because the Temple World was needed as a step to get you to the Field. The Temple World prepares you to ultimately see the Field and connect to the whole. The discoveries you've made have prepared you to see the Field and believe that it's actually there *and* that you're part of it. You're far more extraordinary than you believe you are in everyday reality.

Even though the Field wasn't introduced at the beginning of the Temple Journey, it didn't mean it wasn't at play. It was at play from the very first moment we walked through the entryway. The field of quantum energy took us all the way to the end of this journey, which, as you may be guessing, isn't the end. There is no end. Only infinity. Even when you're not journeying inside the Temple World, you're always inside it.

The same holds true for the people who've passed on. The

only difference is that we can no longer observe their existence in this 3-D reality because they don't have a body—at least, not one as dense as ours. But they're always part of us inside the Temple World. They're always part of the Field. They're always part of our essence and existence. The Field isn't only responsible for the thought-matter interaction; it's also responsible for removing the separation between you and the person you lost.

When we first went through the Door in my class, I did not expect my students to see their beloveds right away, but to my surprise, when everyone returned, all they could talk about was how they'd experienced the presence of their loved ones. I was so surprised that it happened so soon. *How could that be?* I asked myself. And the answer was obvious. The Field was there from the beginning. It connected us to our beloveds from the get-go. It also connected us to each other.

It All Ends Where It Starts

I remember moments after Bjarne passed over, I sat on his bedside looking up at the ceiling, searching for him. I should have known to look not up but to look everywhere. I should have put my hands out, closed my eyes, and felt him filling the entire space between his dead body and my tortured one. He had become everything that stood between us. I just didn't know it.

Now I know why I didn't see anything when I looked up. He wasn't rising, he was expanding. And as I'm writing this to you, in this moment, I can almost feel him surrounding me. He's been waiting a long time for me to arrive here.

The first time I saw the Field, I walked out a newly discovered back door in my Temple and into a field of beautiful flowers, soft grass, and a sun that was perfectly setting—luminous oranges, reds, and purples. (Keep in mind, the Field you see in your journey will be specific to you.) There, in the midst of all this beauty, thousands of people stood waiting for me. I wondered who they were. My best guess was that they were the people who have passed on waiting for their loved ones to come find them. But I barely glanced at them; I was looking for Bjarne. I'd seen him many times during my journeys to the Temple World and thought he would be there waiting for me as I completed this experience. But he wasn't among this sea of people, and you know what? I was okay with that.

I learned along the way that my journey through the Door is much bigger than connecting with him. Much bigger than simply knowing where he's been since his passing. The journey to this place that I named the Temple World holds intelligence that I didn't expect, a collective consciousness, where everything connects. This intelligence holds the concept of time by storing its memories and creations in the present moment. It tracks everything that's ever been and everything that will ever be. It communicates this knowledge in the most subtle but certain ways and does so in an instant. It removes the laws of physicality, the rules of this reality.

When I discovered that this final stop, this interaction with the Field, would be an integral part of the Temple World, I was very eager to take this journey. I couldn't wait. I'd been feeling the pull without knowing what it was since I'd passed through the Door on my very first Temple Journey. The force of the Field urged me in ways I cannot fully articulate. It begged me to enter. It called me at night. It grabbed me by my soul and pulled me inside. As if, well, as if this world beyond the Door were always part of me. Familiar, yet completely unknown until my feet stepped inside the Field.

I felt surrounded by the knowledge of who I am, who I've always been throughout time and space. The Field connected me with all my selves, histories, future selves, and destinies—all these possibilities, these multiple universes, caught up in one wave. I was a body of quantum energy communicating with the sea of people I saw inside my Field. There was information coming to me, specific information about my past—not possibilities of my past, but certainties. I was told that I'd always been a teacher and a writer, that these are my gifts, and that I should never doubt them. The intelligence of the Temple World was coming through loud and clear as I was feeling the force of the Field. My cognition had no boundaries. It moved beyond anything that was linear, logical, and physical. It felt like an ocean of energy, a sea of vibration, that connected me with the entire Temple Journey in an infinite whorl of energy. Infinitely swirling in a circular fashion. Infinitely mine.

The people in the Field were silent but full of the kind of knowledge I needed. My observation of this massive Field of people was enough to spark the knowing. There was a life force that connected me to the Field, connected me to the people—all of whom were strangers to me in my own 3-D reality but seemed familiar as they stood there. They wore kind expressions and held a reverence for me and for all beings—appreciating my willingness to go beyond the container of my world. They knew me, and I knew them. The energetic pull I felt from them didn't feel like love as we know it, but a love that was beyond what we think of as human love. Beyond the ego and boundaries of self that so often get in our way. For me, this love and intelligence came to me through this group of people. Everyone will have their own experience in the Field—there may be only a couple of people in your Field, or a stadium full, or none at all, but everyone who has done this journey has felt that feeling of love and intelligence from the Field.

The Field was forceful but gentle. Surprising but familiar. Astonishing but humble. No ego. Just being. A blueprint of my soul and all souls. I walked farther into the Field, thinking I'd gain more knowledge, but the knowledge was the same wherever I moved. The Field wasn't changing its charge. It was always the same and always enough—a web of equally charged energy. I don't know why the first time I went to my own Field there were thousands of people waiting for me. I started directing my thoughts toward all those people by just feeling their presence. This is hard to articulate. It felt as if the communication were taking place outside of time. And they knew I was feeling the exchange from them for the first time consciously. It didn't even matter who they were, where they came from, and why they were there. What mattered was what I felt. The connection. The knowing. The being with them. The effortless way of communicating. In a way I was them, they were me. We were whole. We were the Field, the Field was us, and we were interacting with each other.

In a sense, I was grateful to have this experience and didn't need to know the why of it. I just felt honored. My view of the world, my world, was changing enough to allow for this experience. At this point I was arriving at a place where I didn't need to back everything up with science. My experiences were enough. I didn't need the validation of science to make me feel that my experience counted. The story I'd been telling myself for years changed. I started to emerge from the Temple World as an ancient and timeless soul. Although I will always believe in science, the fact is that I now believe in myself *more* than science. The ultimate truth is not the result of some experiment that took place fifty years ago, but the truth of what I experience on these journeys, inside the world beyond the Door. My truth.

My relationship with my own life changed even more in this journey, where I went inside the Field. Finally, I viewed my life in this 3-D reality through the Field. I saw myself sitting in my chair, taking this journey. The Field made me feel whole. It was as if I had everything I needed and there was nothing more I wished for. I was enough. I had enough. It connected me with all the versions of me that were scattered in the universe forgotten by my soul. The Field Journey brought them back together. And yet that felt unsettling. "Unsettling" is the word I choose to use here. Even though the Field is the most beautiful space you'll ever enter, its presence is alarming. Being connected to everything and everyone feels a little intrusive to the ego. But as you continue to do the Field Journey, that unsettled feeling evaporates, and the connection to yourself and everything else, the depth and dimensions of who you are, will feel most natural.

The way you observed your life in 3-D is going to magnify

everything that's going to happen this week. Watch and see the miracle-like experiences that will take place because you will be observing with such an intense feeling of joy and happiness. Your increased appreciation of all the goodness you have in your life and the way you experience that will make a tremendous difference. I can't wait to see what this week will bring you.

The Final Journey

Find a comfortable chair in a quiet place where you won't be disturbed. Read the instructions once or twice before you close your eyes to take the journey. Remember to have something on hand—a notebook, an iPad, etc.—to record your experience after the journey. If you'd like, you can play the corresponding sound vibration or other music, or simply proceed in silence. Relax your shoulders. You're in a safe space.

Now we'll journey all the way to the Temple of Universes, along the familiar pathway. This is a journey that builds on itself, so as always, we'll begin with the Door, cross its threshold, connect with your Super Watcher and, together, travel through the Portal and to your Temple.

PART 1. THE FIELD

1. When you arrive at the Temple, step inside. Remain present. Notice each and every detail, noting anything new that's arrived since your last visit. Observe your Miraculous life inside the Temple, the one you've chosen to observe each time you've journeyed there.

2. Look in your Temple Mirror. Notice what you're wearing in your reflection. Is it a beautiful dress? A perfectly tailored suit? Your favorite jeans? Or maybe it's something very different from what you're used to, a style and fabric you've never seen before. What do you look like?

3. Now, you're going to find your way out of the Temple. Whoever you saw in the Mirror, bring him or her outside with you. This time, you'll exit through a Door to the back, opposite where you entered. This is a Door you haven't seen before.

4. There's a Field that surrounds the Temple. Step out into it. Remember, your Field might have orange grass or flying trees, or it might look might look like the aurora borealis, interconnected strings of light, or swirling needles of light.

5. Feel the presence of that continuous field of energy stream through your mind, your thoughts, your body, the Temple, your life, your creations—everything connects to the Field. As you walk through the Field, take everything in—the messages, the visions, the experiences you're having. You begin to feel that you have a bigger destiny and that all versions of yourself are here. Hold on to that feeling.

6. As you make your way through the Field, walk toward your life in your day-to-day reality. Just set your destination and you'll find your way. Trust yourself. Going into your 3-D life

from the Field will feel different from any experiences you've had so far.

7. Here you are. Now walk inside your life. Up ahead, you'll find your home. You'll see yourself in your chair with your eyes closed, taking this journey. Observe yourself. What do you see when you look at yourself? Look around the room. Look at your home. See the people in your life, your thoughts, your errands, your friends, your street, your neighborhood, your town, your job, the places you get to go every day. Witness it all through the eyes of the Field.

8. Find your way back to the Field. See how close it is? Your life and the Temple aren't far apart at all, held closely by the power of the Field. Walk back through the Field, toward the Temple. You're going to enter back through the back Door from which you accessed the Field, but before you walk inside, turn back and take one last look at the Field. This isn't good-bye; this is welcome back. The Field will always be with you.

9. As you walk through the Temple of Universes, the Field is walking with you. The Field is connected to your Super Watcher, who's connected to your physical body. Finally, with your Super Watcher beside you, walk back to the Portal, go through it, through time and space. Bring back with you not only the feelings, insights, purpose, and meaning but everything you captured and the new you that you've become

through this journey. Every journey changes you and elevates you and gets you closer to the person you truly are.

10. Now you're at the Door and it's time to cross back into your 3-D life. Come back to your chair. Take a deep breath. Another deep breath. Now you may open your eyes.

The Yellow Rubber Duckie

I'm going to take you back to the beginning of the journey so you can see how the Field was always in action. The first time I did the Super Watcher Activation Journey with the class it was only the second time we'd met, yet we were connected from the beginning. I didn't realize how connected until our rubber duckie experience. I've been waiting to tell you this story since the beginning of this book.

The object I found to bring back was truly unexpected—a yellow rubber duckie. At the time, I thought, *How will I ever find a rubber duckie in my 3-D life? Where could I possibly stumble upon one? I don't have small kids anymore. I don't have any friends with small kids.* But it was the object I saw, the object I was supposed to bring back with me. Since the idea is not to seek the object but to let it come to you, I had no choice but to wait for the rubber duckie to make its appearance during that next week.

When we regrouped after the journey, I told everyone that my object was the rubber duckie and expressed how impossible I thought it would be to find it. A few others in the class felt their objects were surprising and would be impossible to find as well. I told them that trusting the intelligence of the Temple Journey is part of the experience. The object that appears to us on the other side of the Door isn't from our ego, but from our Super Watcher, which has no ego, no expectations. We don't have to be logical. We just have to trust. We journey every day so that we can learn to switch from our Survivor (ego) to the Super Watcher self inside the Temple of Universes, our Super Watcher, which always serves us best.

The rubber duckie was my object, and I had to trust what I believed to be true—that one day in that next week I'd unexpectedly find it. And I did. Three days after our second class, I opened my folder on my computer to download a document, and there it was, in plain sight. A rubber duckie stuck on top of the Word file icon. I had never seen it before, but this folder had been there for a really long time. I immediately signed into our online class community to share that I'd found my object, how I'd found it, and where.

Within a few hours, something amazing started to happen and continued for months. One by one, nearly everyone in class—close to fifty students—started finding rubber duckies in their lives. Not just one duckie per person, but multiple duckies. The yellow rubber duckies filled our community forum. Participants found them in the most unexpected places—inside their swimming pool, at the dentist, on top of cars, inside their brand-new hot tubs, in the bank, and on and on.

This was a big deal because once my object was brought into the Field, every person inside the Field of the class was also connected to it. And it kept materializing in their own day-to-day lives. On top of that, other people's objects—for example, the key, the purple ball of yarn, a coin, a rock were also being discovered by their classmates. This class, what we were experiencing and exploring together on the other side of the Door, deepened our connection. We were observing each other's realities. We weren't self-contained, separate lives. We were connected.

And if that's true, then when our loved ones move on, we are still linked to them, and when we do so also, we remain connected to everyone and everything. All I want to do for you with this book is to show you that you live inside a big universe in which everything—whether it's visible to you or not—is connected. And you can connect to anyone in the whole world. I still see rubber duckies everywhere I go. So do the participants in the class. I believe we'll always see them. The rubber duckies now live in our Field with us.

Your Homework for This Week

Now think about the incredible life you observed on the other side of the Door. Your observing it will bring it to life. The Field does that. There's a dynamic interaction at play at all times. Your daily journeys allow you to experience that interaction and help you to consciously play with it. This week, to deepen your experience of the Field, focus on the points below.

OBSERVE THE MESSAGES FROM THE FIELD

As you're traveling through the Field, let your thoughts interact with the energy. You're always interacting anyway. Observe your interactions. What thoughts are going into the Field and what is generated in your 3 D life from what you have observed in the Field? These observations will begin to take shape in your reality, appearing as visions, or as thoughts, or as eagerness for action. Be mindful of that.

DISCOVER THE SPECIFIC MESSAGE ABOUT YOUR CURRENT LIFE IN THE 3-D WORLD

What did you discover from the Field? What did you observe in going back to your house through the eyes of the Field? Write your observations down in great detail. Every time you journey to the Field, connect to the vibration of it. Become one. And then come back to this reality. What do you see differently? What's there that you couldn't see before?

NOTICE WHAT'S CHANGING IN YOUR LIFE

Observe what's happening in your everyday reality. There are tiny changes that need observing. The more you observe these changes the more real they become. The Field removes the separation between "I" and "this." Your Temple World, your new life, what you see inside are all one with you.

The way we're most accustomed to creating a new reality is with action. Now you can take action toward bringing the Temple World in this 3-D reality. For example, if or when you encounter the dress you saw in the Mirror, buy it, buy the curtains, the flowers. If you see a partner in the Temple World, write about him or her in your journal. Paint what you see. And continue to be open to the flow of miracles, to the objects and experiences that show up without you doing anything about them.

Now that you've seen your new reality through the eyes of the Field, write in detail anything and everything that come your way. Write it out and share with someone in your life or pair up in your Temple Circle, or get on a Skype call to share your new life. The details, the feelings, all of it. You have now experienced the Temple World many times. It's time to be very clear about your life ahead. To do that, focus on what the Field is telling you about your purpose and meaning in this life. The more you visit, the stronger the connection. The more you believe in the Field interaction, the more the Field will interact with you. Your ability to create and connect with the world beyond the Door will increase each time you visit. You are expanding the world of possibilities for your life.

8

welcome

Deep down the consciousness of mankind is one. . . .
if we don't see this, it's because we are blinding ourselves to it.
—JOSEPH RIGGIO

These days, I enter through the Door to the Temple World as casually as I walk through the front door of my house. It's that natural. Yet, unlike the door to my house, which remains predictably the same, each time I begin a journey the Door to the Temple World changes, depending on what's taking place in my life. When I'm feeling nostalgic or sad, the Door might appear old, with worn, polished wood. If I'm excited about the journey ahead, it might be large, covered in multicolored glitter. I've never seen the exact same Door twice, and I've never had the same journey—each one is different, the gifts I bring back are different, the new visions for my life and the wisdom I gain are unique.

I'm especially eager to visit when I am struggling to see my life with more clarity. On those days, I go through the Door to find comfort in being with my Super Watcher—because she knows on a deep level how unbreakable I am, and reminds me of that the moment we meet. No words pass between us, but when I'm in her presence, I feel that I deeply know my eternal cosmic self—a wiser, older, timeless part of me. After I depart the Temple World, my Super Watcher remains with me for a while, helping me to be faster, smarter, wiser.

I started this journey to find Bjarne. While I continue to visit him in the Temple World, and I love seeing him there, he is no longer the only reason for the visit. Now we're both a little more distant. It's as if he knows I no longer need him as I did when I started this work. He knows I received what I was supposed to receive. I can see him smiling as I write these words. He knew this journey was more about my life than about his death. He knew from the beginning that I was seeking to find a better life for myself outside of the Survivor self and the constraints of this 3-D life. Of course, it's always nice to see him, but I have other relationships inside my Temple World that I experience as well.

I especially love to see my guides. This is one of the most warm and comforting experiences of my current physical life. As soon as I enter the Door, there they are, waiting, excited. When I haven't visited in a few days I tend to fall back into my Survivor self and become more vulnerable to my fears, of which I have quite a few. My guides—there are two of them—seem eager, every time, to get me through the Door, communicating their feelings telepathically, asking, *What took you so long?* They console me, soothe my day-to-day stress. Each holds one of my hands as we walk toward the Temple of Universes, and they remind me that all's well in the world. All's well with me. They smile, they sparkle, they beam with joy. It's the joy I feel when I pass through the Door that fills me with a deep knowing that this is not a fantasy, not my imagination. You can't feel this kind of joy and bliss when you're imagining things. Not to this extent, anyway, this overwhelming wave of bliss, a knowing, a calm that comes with being one with all.

I am always shocked that I discovered happiness on the path I built to find Bjarne. Losing him caused me so much pain, I knew I had to find closure. I was determined. But this experience has brought so much more than closure, so much more than I could have imagined; it has gone beyond healing. I didn't expect to come face-to-face with my inner bliss. I didn't know others would, too. My religious upbringing emphasized heaven as a reward for living a moral life, but I was also hugely influenced by the prospect of a possible hell, that dark world full of unknown entities. In the church of my earlier life, death was feared and, of course, the place behind the veil has, accordingly, always been a little scary to me.

The science of consciousness provided me with a path to explore what follows death that didn't include fear. Because of science—quantum mechanics, particle physics, neuroscience—I was able to discover the universe awaiting me behind the Door. It's very hard to be afraid of atoms, particles, and scientific words, isn't it? When science proves the seemingly impossible it quiets our emotions and fears. The traditional ghosts and spirits of the underworld are replaced with possibilities.

Even though grounding myself in science gave me the courage to open the Door to the Temple World, and took me partway to the Temple of Universes, it was my own experiences that made me a believer in this place we mistakenly call "the afterlife." The world beyond the Door is not the afterlife. What lies within the Temple

World is so much more than an "after" experience. Within the Temple World is our whole existence, our every memory, every journey. This life we live in our day-to-day reality is such a small piece of what takes place outside the physical boundaries and walls we've created within our conscious bodies. It can be frightening, or at least unsettling, to think that our lives are in truth larger than what happens between before and after. But it's true.

Every Temple Journey Changes You

Each journey I take changes me. The truths I discover shift my thoughts. I experience myself outside my body, outside the physical space I inhabit. Because of that, my body has changed, my energy has changed, and my identity has changed (and all continue to do so), incorporating more fully the essence of all the selves I've ever had. For every time I look at myself in the Temple Mirror, I see another me who lives, lived, or will live in timelessness outside my day-to-day reality.

Every time I go through the Door I gain part of me that's been missing. It's not that I become new; rather, I grow older. Older, deeper, and wiser than I ever imagined. Where I once felt fear—of death, the invisible world beyond this one—I now feel excitement about visiting that world, the possibilities it holds. Sure, my brain still tries to go back to the old routine of small, constraining beliefs—that death is real and that our abilities are limited—but when I feel I'm getting caught up in that way of thinking, I sit down, close my eyes, visit the Temple World, and seek my many selves. I feel the bliss of being in a place outside the trauma, loss, and stark so-called reality of our third-dimensional world.

And when I visit my husband, I make new memories with him. How do you make memories with someone who's passed? How do you do that and still consider yourself a sane person? But I do have new memories—of seeing Bjarne inside the Temple World, guiding me through the Portal, walking with me to the Temple of Universes. My daughter Isabel has also made new memories with her dad. And that is one thing I never thought could be possible. If you told me eleven years ago that my daughter would be creating new memories with her dad after his passing I never would have believed it—and I would have laughed out loud at the thought.

One of my favorite new memories of Bjarne is of the very first time I saw him on the other side of the Door. He was sitting at a café, and as soon as he saw me, he asked me to bring the girls to him. Immediately, and surprisingly, the girls showed up. I know you are aware by now that this is the kind of thing that happens inside the Temple World, but at the time I was astonished. No words were uttered. We all hugged for the first time in years. When I shared this part of my visit with my girls, they shared with me their own new memories of their dad from their journeys. As you know, I've taken the girls on the journey to the Temple World many times. They've met their Super Watchers. They've met their dad. It's easier for kids to go beyond the Door to the Temple World. They have fewer boundaries than adults. They're freer to believe in what they cannot see, freer to believe in the afterlife, the life beyond our third dimension.

I know you purchased this book to find out where your loved one had gone. And as it turns out, you traveled outside time and space not only to find him or her, but also to find the truth about your own existence—and to create that existence. Remember, the more you visit the Temple World, the more you will connect to the invisible field that is your partner in the dance of cocreation.

The world beyond coexists with this world, but few choose to see it. Our ability to see that world and play with it changes not only the way we live life after loss but also how we live life. Period. We enter cosmic consciousness. Activating your cosmic self (your Super Watcher) changes your everyday life in ways you can't imagine and others might not understand. You won't get so wound up by the drama of day-to-day life. You'll view and speak of death differently. You'll be living a life not driven by fear.

This new perspective on life and death will place you in the minority when it comes to how we, collectively, view what is "real." But one day soon, I believe many more people will join us. Awareness is increasing on the planet. People are waking up. Accessing and harnessing the truth about our soul are our birthrights. Death is real in our world because we're observing its realness. But when we observe the Temple World and experience new, undeniable moments of truth, we will observe death very differently. We will have no choice but to accept this new truth—that we're more in control of the possibilities life offers us than we thought, and that we never lose the people we love. We lose them only in this dimension, but in every other dimension, our loves are regained.

The Journey: It's More About Creation Than Grief

From now on, spending some time outside our 3-D reality will be a necessity for you. You must aim to spend ten minutes each day in the Temple World, accessing the divine intelligence that leads you to the observations that serve your life here and beyond. And, of course, to spend time with your loved ones if you wish to. As time goes by, they'll show themselves to you less and less because they know that you're in this physical world to live in the physical world. This message came across loud and clear when I was teaching the class and writing this book. As the class went on, the participants spent less time with their loved ones and more time understanding reality in this new way through the Temple World. I was surprised and thrilled to see how quickly the Temple Journey work moved them forward from their grief. And I know you've probably experienced the same thing. You're experiencing such growth and joy, you're embracing life not because you've stopped loving the one who has passed on, but because the natural way of life is to find a path forward, reaching toward peace and bliss rather than toward the past. The ones we lost offer us a bridge, not a destination.

The question I asked in the beginning of this book—"Where did you go?"—was just the first step toward a journey unlike anything else, a journey not just about finding our beloveds, but also about finding ourselves and figuring out the bigger things in life. Finding the courage to expand our experiences beyond the traditional horizon of the world we live in.

It takes guts to embrace the vastness and the powers of your consciousness while grieving the loss of someone you love so deeply. But that's exactly the time we must do it. The death of someone we loved shifts reality as we have known it. This wrenching shift, as terrible as it is, brings us to a unique emotional and psychological moment in our lives—a moment when reality is up for question; a moment when we are open to surrendering to something profound yet invisible; a moment when at any other time we may not even be capable of considering the possibility of a cosmic identity. The death of a loved one brings forth an opening just wide enough for us to squeeze in and seek our own truth, to seek the multidimensional world where you will find your beloved. You want to be part of it. You want to go inside this place your beloved has gone, reach for their hand, and let them give you a hug. And in that reaching, you find not just them but also the place from which you've come, the place where you belong.

The Temple Journey reminds you of the power and dimensions that live within you and opens you to a new way of living in this world. Your entryway doesn't just take you closer to the person you lost, it also takes you closer to your own timeless consciousness. Away from form but closer to the source of form. Closer to creation. And above all, closer to the divinity of the soul.

It's easy to look at the world and see its physical nature, get caught up in the material, the concrete, the business, the supposed logic. But it becomes increasingly difficult to continue seeing it like this when you've spent time exploring synchronicities, miracles, communications with people you've lost, and the creation of your physical world from inside your consciousness. Then you realize that the world you see isn't physical and mindless, but formless and full of awareness. You discover that your mind can create matter in a beautiful, serene way. You experience peace and bliss unlike anything you've felt.

Your Super Watcher started as a way to help you distance yourself from your thoughts and from the material world when you crossed through the entryway. It was there to take you by the hand and walk with you inside an unfamiliar world. It was there to show you how to detach from your body and fly away free. It was there very purposefully. As you've taken the journeys in this book and done your homework, you've mostly likely become aware of the change in your Super Watcher. As you evolved, you became more aware of its vastness. It became the entire universe with everything inside it. It was the entire Temple World. It became the Field, the Portal, and the Door. And since the Super Watcher is also you, you became the universe, the Temple of Universes, the Field, the Portal, and the Door. Do you see how you're connected to everything?

My intention is for you to learn to trust your experiences enough to believe that you belong in two worlds— the physical, temporary one and the nonphysical, infinite one. These two worlds are connected by the Door, which bridges the divide. My hope is that you have experienced enough connection, miracles, and synchronicity in our time together in these pages that you'll keep going deeper.

We Visit Them; They're Not Visiting Us

One of the very first things I learned on this journey was that those we've lost didn't just want us to visit them, they also wanted us to recognize our ability to create our life, to discover the connection points of the two worlds and master them. I experienced this myself; I saw this with my class. The thirst for creating new life was greater than the pull toward living in the past.

Our soul yearns to connect with the timeless and invisible world without having to physically die. The lessons we learn from an awakened state are much greater than the lessons we learn from our limited, fear-based, physical world. What we bring back from that limitless world can help us expand this one. Can help us bring beauty and joy into our everyday lives. Grief is also a fear of being without the ones we loved. The Temple World replaces that fear with peace, changing your reality and the routine of your daily life as you witness miracles becoming everyday occurrences.

I hope you now realize that the way we see our life influences the way we evolve as human beings. I want you to start seeing everything through the filter of the Temple World, where everything exists forever, where all that is lives outside time and space, and where death is not real. This is your birthright. The Temple Journey is a map I've created to take you inside your own human evolution so we can all start taking steps forward and create a reality without death, without end, and without limitations. I do know this is probably scary to some, and in many ways, it should be.

If we believe that our perception of reality is the only boundary between ourselves and infinity, then the responsibility of infinity is one not to be taken lightly. We can see that we will need to be careful that our thoughts are creating positive futures. The next frontier is not the exploration of space but the exploration into consciousness, where everything is yours for the taking. Your dreams. Your passions. Your desired life. But it requires one thing. Belief. Belief that it's possible. Belief that even though the person you loved exited this physical plane, they're very much alive inside a cosmic consciousness that is of a piece and one with the infinite universe.

When the Physical Reality Pulls You Away from the Nonphysical

I know your day-to-day life can keep you busy and away from the Temple World, but it's important to make the time. You'll find the journey brings you back to your higher self, your divinity, and the cosmos. You'll ease the doubts that can creep in when your senses are bombarded by the material world, when you get caught up in the illusion of this world. But ultimately, it's not so much that the journey will lessen your doubts, but that your Super Watcher will come along with you in this reality, too. And the more objects, experiences, and images you find in this dimension that you first encountered in the Temple Journey, the more you'll know that what you experienced was not a fantasy. The more you'll receive wisdom and clarity from the Temple World, the more your life here will change.

I did not write this book to introduce you to a meditation process. The Temple Journey is not a meditation. Absolutely not. I do not seek to guide you into the nothingness of consciousness. I seek to take you into the vastness of a complex universe and show you that you are not only part of it, not only an observer, but that you are also the creator. I want to bring you friends; community; and new, fulfilling experiences. I want to give you the tools to mend your heart one small step at a time and reconnect you with those you lost. To show you that, actually, you never lost them. The Field is everywhere. The Temple World is inside you, and outside. And your beloved is and always will be part of your consciousness, part of the stars in your sky, the cosmos. Your loved one is inside the Field where you exist right now. You can give them form when you go inside the Temple World and see them, talk to them, be with them. You can give form to your thoughts and dreams and participate in creating a reality you want inside the hologram. After all, it has always been you. You are the one who got us here, inside this book. Inside the Temple World. You created it for yourself, and you brought me into your life to share it with you. The Temple World is our creation.

I have tears in my eyes thinking of what a gift this will be for the rest of your life. This Temple Journey is going to be part of you forever. The Door, the Portal, and the house of creation that is the Temple of Universes. Ultimately, the Temple World will be living inside you and you'll have access to it every day. Almost like a prayer. A place of complete transcendence.

Where to Next?

So, what comes next? How do you bring the Temple World into your day-to-day life, since it is this 3-D world you're meant to be living in now? And how is this all going to continue to make you feel more aware, more whole, and more a part of a bigger universe? I'm grateful for your many crossings and journeys since you opened the pages of this book. I am grateful for where you have arrived. Living your life knowing that it is so much bigger than it seems, with so much more possibility than most people know. And above all that death is not real outside of this physical plane.

As for me, I'm no longer afraid of the dark, of ghosts, and of the energy that lives outside of this 3-D reality. If certain experiences and people enter my life that must mean that I created them. I now know I'm not just the observer but also the participator (and so are you). That in and of itself makes the unseen less frightening, and my future, too.

Going forward, the most important thing is to journey ten minutes each day if you can. The journeys to the Temple World allow for your participation in your creation to become conscious instead of accidental. More focused instead of miraculous and rare. The journeys bring back peace, joy, and a grounding that isn't possible without traveling outside the physical reality with our consciousness. However, the journeys don't bring back the dead. Instead, the dead take you to where they now live. For me, that's good enough.

What we truly wish for is less loneliness: to feel connected to someone or something bigger than ourselves. We wish for mastery of our lives after loss, participation in our destiny. And that's what the Temple World is here to provide. Participation in this life, creation of our destiny, and connection to those we lost from this world. You may question everything even after experiencing as much as you have. That's okay. This is the nature of evolution and exploration. In grief, we must question. In mourning, we must seek to find. And in being stuck, we must get up and boldly travel to where we have never been before.

Now that you've seen the path, you make the path yours. Now that you've taken all the steps, you dance instead of walk. Fly instead of run. And you look in the Mirror, open to all the extraordinary facets of your Super Watcher. It's time to acknowledge that you're not just infinite, but also multidimensional. You're not just formless, but also the form you created. You're the warrior who transforms into a monk, and the monk who transforms into a warrior. You are everything you can be. You are the Temple World.

acknowledgments

Where Did You Go? was born of my need to fly farther from my safety net. If it weren't for my husband, Eric, who's always believed in me, I may not have soared as high as I have. My daughters, Elina and Isabel, who said a big yes to the Temple World from the beginning. I knew that if I created this journey just so they could meet their dad it would be more than worth it.

My parents, Niko and Despina, who despite the expectations of everyone in the small Greek town I was raised in— that I would marry and settle down—gave me permission to open my wings and fly inside a Temple World I could not yet see. My sister, Artemis, for always loving me and supporting me over the years. Thank you.

I could not have dared to go beyond the world of brain science and into the world of consciousness if my literary agent, Stephanie Tade, hadn't looked me in the eye and said, "This is the book you want to write, and this is the book you should write." Without that moment of a big yes from her it may have taken me much longer to embrace the Temple World.

My gratitude for the incredible team at HarperOne, who saw the book for what it was from the very first moment we met. Thank you to my beautiful editor at HarperOne, Libby Edelson, for her passion and love for my work. I felt so safe with you. When I sent the book in I knew you would find all the places I couldn't see and help me light them up. For sitting by my side for so many days toward the end going over every single word with me.

Kelly Malone, for editing me while loving my voice, for helping me see the rhythm in my words, and for putting up with me during all the stressful times I couldn't see this book the way you could. And for reminding me that the beauty of this book was there from the beginning.

Claudia Boutote, for saying such a big yes to this book from the very first time we met.

Eva Avery, so grateful for your love for the book.

My Life Reentry Institute team, who work day in and day out to keep the institute growing. Carole Marie, Justin, Eduardo, Christy—who make my work fly across the globe every single day, I'm forever grateful for you. Jeff Suburu, for recording the Temple World Sound Frequency and for taking all my messy instructions and bringing back vibrational sounds that felt so right.

My soul sisters Jenny Thompson, Erin Matlock, Leanne Ely, Zeta Pappastrati, Shannon Amsler Nigro, Nathalie, Dolisy Lecluse, Joanne Sheriff Todd, Kristine Carlson, Allison Maslan, Elaine Glass and Michelle Steinke Baumgard. I love being on this journey with all of you.

Charlie Gilkey, for walking with me even though my steps were all over the place. I thank you for always reminding me I am no longer the underdog. Michael Fishman, for always seeing my light before anyone else did. Michael Margolis, for being on this amazing journey with me. Robin Seemangal, for being my Star Letters partner and loving rockets as much as I do. Amelie de Mahy, for keeping my body in the right frequency with her on-point acupuncture needles throughout the year of this book. Dr. Anne Gartner, for helping my body find its way back. Dr. Guillermo Ruiz, for walking by my side toward a healthier future. Anastasia Rivas, for making me always feel beautiful in your chair. Franco Maccarthy, for taking chances with my hair all year long. With the help you all gave, I transitioned to a new physical reality.

And to the first Temple Journeyers in our pilot Beyond Reentry class who said yes to this journey before this book was written and before anyone ever heard of the Temple World. I could not have done it without you. And finally to my dogs, Tyson and Gracie, for keeping me company as I sat at my desk writing this book.

resources

To evolve to a place of a basic understanding of the universe we must spend time delving into a world of knowledge about what the cosmos is made of. Without these resources, I could not have written this book or found my way into the Temple World. Our everyday lives are made of many 3-D images. Seeing from a different place will allow you to create and live a life of joy and miracles after loss. If you haven't lost someone and want to live life more fully, you'll also be able to live a joy-filled, miraculous life. Life after loss, life in general, shouldn't be as hard as it is. And remember, always trust that the Temple World is as real as everything you see, touch, and connect with around you.

Online Support with This Book

- Temple World Sounds. Here is where you can easily download the sound for your journeys: https://lifereentry.com/templevibration.com/.

- ChristinaRasmussen.com. Stop by my main home—Christina Rasmussen's Universe.

- LifeReentry.com. Search for online or offline Temple Circles and upcoming classes at the Life Reentry Institute

- Private Facebook Group Where Did You Go?: https://www.facebook.com/groups/wheredidyougo/.
- SecondFirsts.com. Find articles of inspiration after loss.
- StarLetters.com. Born out of my own passion for rockets, stars, space news, and consciousness evolution, I created this site, which is dedicated to outer space, rocket launches, and consciousness.

Online Resources about the Cosmos

- DiscoverMagazine.com. Mind & Brain, Space & Physics, Technology—an incredible resource for all curious minds.
- NASA.gov. I visit this site almost daily to read about new missions and space exploration.
- ScientificAmerican.com. This is one of my favorite magazines to learn about new discoveries in space and on our planet Earth.
- Space.com. Learn all about what's up with outer space, space travel, and the latest technology—everything from artificial intelligence to the supersonic parachutes created for the Mars landing.

Books I Love About the Universe

Each book in this category brings forth an element of truth about the universe we live in. It always strikes me as strange that we don't know much about our universe and how we interact with it. Without you there would be no universe. And without the universe there would be no you. The dance I mentioned in the book—between you and the universe, you and the Field—happens inside all these books. Read on. Dance away . . .

Deepak Chopra. *The Seven Spiritual Laws of Success: A Practical Guide for the Fulfillment of Your Dreams* and *You Are the Universe: Discovering Your Cosmic Self and Why It Matters.*

Brian Greene. *The Hidden Reality: Parallel Universes and the Deep Laws of the Cosmos.*

Stephen Hawking. *A Brief History of Time: And Other Essays.*

Robert Lanza. *Beyond Biocentrism: Rethinking Time, Space Consciousness, and the Illusion of Death.*

Lynne McTaggart. *The Field: The Quest for the Secret Force of the Universe.*

Michael Talbot. *The Holographic Universe: The Revolutionary Theory of Reality* and *Mysticism and the New Physics.*

Life-Changing Books About Cocreating with the Universe

Bruce Lipton, Wayne Dyer, Esther Hicks, and many more write about the powers we have inside us that can almost seem like a magic wand. Something so fairy tale–like that our logical brain doesn't want to believe it. If nothing else, this book proved to you that cocreating with the universe is no tale.

Gregg Braden. *The Divine Matrix: Bridging Time, Space, Miracles, and Belief.*

Dr. Joe Dispenza. *You Are the Placebo: Making Your Mind Matter.*

Mike Dooley. *Choose Them Wisely: Thoughts Become Things!*

Wayne W. Dyer, PhD. *Change Your Thoughts—Change Your Life: Living the Wisdom of the Tao.*

Pam Grout. *E-Squared: Nine Do-It-Yourself Energy Experiments That Prove Your Thoughts Create Your Reality.*

Esther Hicks and Jerry Hicks. *Ask and It Is Given: Learning to Manifest Your Desires* and *The Law of Attraction: The Basics of the Teachings of Abraham.*

Napoleon Hill. *Think and Grow Rich.*

Bruce H. Lipton, PhD. *The Biology of Belief 10th Anniversary Edition: Unleashing the Power of Consciousness, Matter & Miracles.*

Helen Schucman and Robert Perry. *A Course in Miracles.*

Gary Zukav. *The Seat of the Soul.*

My Favorite Books About the Afterlife

I've always been fascinated by the afterlife, but most books don't do it justice. Along with *Where Did You Go?* please also read these books. They'll provide substance, detail, and above all further understanding about the place we call the beyond.

Eben Alexander III MD. *Proof of Heaven: A Neurosurgeon's Journey into the Afterlife.*

Raymond Moody. *Life After Life: The Bestselling Original Investigation That Revealed "Near-Death Experiences."*

Claire Bidwell Smith. *After This: When Life Is Over, Where Do We Go?*

Brian L. Weiss. *Many Lives, Many Masters: The True Story of a Prominent Psychiatrist, His Young Patient, and the Past-Life Therapy That Changed Both Their Lives.*

Books About Awakening I Read and Reread

In the past few years we've seen how the world has started to rise out of darkness and into the light. Even when it seems the darkness has increased, it's simply stronger light shining on what's always been there. These books can help with and support your rise in consciousness. Awakening is more about the resilience to go forth than waking up. We are awake, but now we need to stay awake and to continue tapping into, generating, and spreading the light. And above all, to help others with their process and their journey.

Paolo Coelho. *The Alchemist.*

Osho. *Courage: The Joy of Living Dangerously.*

Michael A. Singer. *The Untethered Soul: The Journey Beyond Yourself.*

Eckhart Tolle. *A New Earth: Awakening to Your Life's Purpose* and *The Power of Now: A Guide to Spiritual Enlightenment.*

the temple circle
getting started guide

A Temple Circle is a group of people who come together each week during the time they're reading *Where Did You Go?* The purpose is for circle members to share their journeys of what took place inside the Temple World. I highly recommend joining a Temple Circle—online or offline—to support you on your journey. My class participants supported each other during the class, and now that we've completed the class, many have continued to meet for continuing growth and support. As you'll discover, the Temple World is a place you visit beyond the reading of this book. Please see the end of this guide to learn how to create a group or join one.

The Observer Effect of the Temple Circle

Nothing in this world exists without an observer. Nothing is created without a witness to the creation. You are the observer, the witness, the seer. And you project your reality into the world and make it 3-D. In other words, you get to determine which universe to create in 3-D. Temple Circles are for those who journey frequently and understand the power of the observer effect. As members (assuming the role of journeyer) share their experiences, the others in the circle assume the role of observers of the journey. The journeys that are shared each week will give the participants who shared the journey validation, support, and acknowledgment of what they experienced. The Temple Circle observer effect will help connect the Temple World with the 3-D world for each journeyer.

The Temple Circle Facilitator

Each week, one journeyer is chosen to become the facilitator for that meeting. The group can choose the facilitator the week before, the day of the meeting, or members can take turns. However, they want to do it. The facilitator leads the group through the journey and makes sure each participant has a chance to share their journey of choice with the Temple Circle. For example, for the Door Journey, members may share any one of the seven journeys they take that week.

Weekly Temple Circle Structure

Each week, the meeting follows the same format.

1. PHYSICAL WORLD CLEANSE

The facilitator starts the meeting with a quick circle version of the Physical World Cleanse, where each member cleanses just one feeling. Going around the circle, each member says, "I feel X." For example, "I feel doubt." "I feel disbelief." "I feel embarrassed to mention this group to my friends." This statement is followed by these words: "Today I cleanse X from my consciousness."

2. THE COLLECTIVE JOURNEY

The facilitator leads the group in a collective journey from that week's chapter—for example, the Door, the Super Watcher Activation, the Mirror. The purposes of the collective journey are for circle members to bond while visiting the Temple World together, and through that bond, to strengthen that experience.

3. SHARING AND OBSERVING THE JOURNEY

Upon finishing the journey and returning to the physical world, members will discuss their experience and observe the experience together. Members share something from that journey or from one of their most memorable journeys from that week, including how their Temple World connected with their physical world.

Some questions members ask themselves or address when speaking about the connection between the two worlds might be:

1. Did you find an object from the Temple World in the physical world?
2. Did your feelings of joy and peace stay with you longer than they have so far?
3. Has your physical experience changed at all? For example, are you walking differently? Did you change how you do your hair?
4. Are your friends noticing anything different about you?
5. Did you come across a building or a familiar image in your physical reality that you saw in your Temple World?

4. REVIEW THAT WEEK'S HOMEWORK ASSIGNMENT

Incorporate the homework at the end of that week's chapter, going through the exercises as a group.

Once everyone has finished the book, it's important to keep meeting. Each meeting will continue to hold the same structure of (1) physical cleanse, (2) collective journey, and (3) sharing and observing. Instead of addressing the homework, you can ask some of the Temple Circle discussion points below. I also encourage you to get creative and develop a structure that works best for your group.

Temple Circle Discussion Points

These discussions are meant to allow for a shift in your general evolution of how you see the physical reality around you, how you now perceive the invisible world beyond the Door, how your life and awareness has shifted, and how your grief has changed.

1. What did you already know about the afterlife before you read *Where Did You Go?*

2. How was *Where Did You Go?* different from those books? What stood out the most that has changed your life more than anything else?

3. Do you feel that *Where Did You Go?* can change the conversation around the afterlife? If yes, how?

4. How did you feel the first time you met with your beloved or your guide?

5. How real does the Temple World feel to you? Do you doubt its realness?

6. Have you read much written about this topic before? If so, does the author bring something unique to the subject?

7. How has this book changed your beliefs about death?

8. How has this book helped you with your grief?

9. Are you connecting with the subject matter? Does it make you want to read more? Does it make you uncomfortable?

10. Is there a chapter or passage that stands out for you or has prompted an aha! moment about the topic?

11. How has finding your first object outside the Temple World influenced your experience of your journeys?

12. How has this book changed your perspective—or maybe even your life? Is that change continuing after reading this book? How?

13. Which part of the Temple World is your favorite?

14. Where do you spend most of your time? Which location in the Temple World?

notes

CHAPTER 1

1. Abraham Maslow, *Religions, Values, and Peak Experiences* (Berlin: Important Books, 2014), pp. 19–29.

CHAPTER 2

1. Lynne McTaggart, *The Field: The Quest for the Secret Force of the Universe* (New York: HarperPerennial, 2012), p. xiii.
2. Michael Talbot, *The Holographic Universe: The Revolutionary Theory of Reality* (New York: HarperPerennial, 2011), p. 53.
3. Melinda Cemira Maxfield, PhD, "Effects of Rhythmic Drumming on EEG and Subjective Experience" (PhD diss., *Institute of Transpersonal Psychology*, 1990), pp. 1–2.

CHAPTER 3

1. Bob Berman and Robert Lanza, *Biocentrism: How Life and Consciousness Are the Keys to Understanding the True Nature of the Universe* (Dallas: BenBella Books, 2010), p. 114.
2. Bernard Haisch, *The God Theory: Universes, Zero-Point Fields, and What's Behind It All* (San Francisco: Red Wheel/Weiser, 2006), pp. 36–37.
3. Berman and Lanza, *Biocentrism*, p. 104.
4. Berman and Lanza, *Biocentrism*, pp. 177–78.
5. Raymond Moody, *Paranormal: My Life in Pursuit of the Afterlife* (New York: HarperOne, 2013), p. 245.

CHAPTER 4

1. "Study reveals substantial evidence of holographic universe," *University of Southampton*, January 31, 2017, https://www.southampton.ac.uk/news/2017/01/holographic-universe.page.
2. Brian Greene, "A Theory of Everything?" *NOVA*, October 28, 2003, http://www.pbs.org/wgbh/nova/physics/theory-of-everything.html/.
3. Michael Talbot, *The Holographic Universe* (New York: HarperPerennial, 1992), pp. 265–66.
4. "Consciousness is tied to 'entropy,' researchers say," *PhysicsWorld*, October 18, 2016, https://physicsworld.com/a/consciousness-is-tied-to-entropy-say-researchers/.

CHAPTER 5

1. Dark Energy, Dark Matter," *NASA Science Beta:* https://science.nasa.gov/astrophysics/focus-areas/what-is-dark-energy.
2. Matt Williams, "A Universe of 10 Dimensions," *Universe Today:* https://www.universetoday.com/48619/a-universe-of-10-dimensions/.
3. Bob Berman and Robert Lanza, "The Biocentric Universe Theory: Life Creates Time, Space, and the Cosmos Itself," Discovermagazine.com, http://discovermagazine.com/2009/may/01-the-biocentric-universe-life-creates-time-space-cosmos.
4. Braden, *The Isaiah Effect*, pp. 100–101.
5. Watts, *Book on the Taboo Against Knowing Who You Are*, p. 130.

CHAPTER 6

1. Charles F. Haanel, *The Master Key System* (New York: SoHo Press, 2013), p. 59.
2. Brian Greene, "A Theory of Everything?" *NOVA*, October 28, 2003, http://www.pbs.org/wgbh/nova/physics/theory-of-everything.html/.
3. Bohn, *Wholeness and Implicate Order*, p. xi.
4. "Quantum Theory and the Uncertainty Principle," *The Physics of the Universe*, https://www.physicsoftheuniverse.com/topics_quantum_nonlocality.html.
5. George Musser, "How Einstein Revealed the Universe's Strange 'Nonlocality,'" *Scientific American*, 2015, https://www.scientificamerican.com/article/how-einstein-revealed-the-universe-s-strange-nonlocality/.
6. Amanda Gefter, "The Case Against Reality," *The Atlantic*, April 25, 2016, https://www.theatlantic.com/science/archive/2016/04/the-illusion-of-reality/479559.

7. Gregg Braden, *Secrets of the Lost Mode of Prayer: The Hidden Power of Beauty, Blessing, Wisdom, and Hurt* (New York: Hay House, 2016), p. 8.
8. P. D. Ouspensky and G. I. Gurdjieff, *In Search of the Miraculous: Fragments from an Unknown Teaching* (New York: Mariner Books, 2001).

CHAPTER 7

1. "Atomic Theory," *Info Please,* https://www.infoplease.com/science-health/physical-science/atomic-theory
2. Mara Johnson-Groh, "NASA listens in as electrons whistle while they work," *Phys.Org,* https://phys.org/news/2017–07-nasa-electrons.html.
3. Mark Pilkington, "Zero Point Energy," *The Guardian,* https://www.theguardian.com/education/2003/jul/17/research.highereducation.
4. McTaggart, *The Field*, p. 96.
5. McTaggart, *The Field*, p. xx.